UNDISCIPLINED HEART

UNDISCIPLINED HEART
Jane Katjavivi

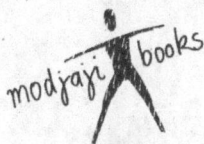

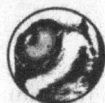

modjaji books

Tigereye

Publication © Modjaji Books 2010
Text © Jane Katjavivi 2010

First published in 2010 by Modjaji Books CC
P O Box 385, Athlone, 7760, South Africa
modjaji.books@gmail.com
http://modjaji.book.co.za

ISBN 978-1-920397-04-3

Namibian edition by Tigereye Publishing
P O Box 24149, Windhoek, Namibia
tigereyepublishing@gmail.com

ISBN: 978-99945-71-06-2

Book design: Natascha Mostert
Cover artwork: Diane Swartzberg
Lettering: Hannah Morris

Printed and bound by Creda Communications, Cape Town
Set in Garamond

To the women I've grown with,
who've shared my life in Namibia,
and who sustain me.

CONTENTS

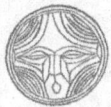

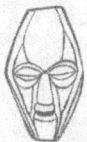

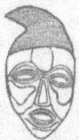

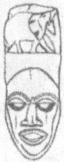

'The mountains do not pray; they are already a part of God's prayers.
They have found their place in the world and here they will stay.
They were here before people looked to the heavens, heard thunder,
and wondered who had created all of this.
We are born, we suffer, we die, and the mountains endure.'

Paulo Coelho
By the River Piedra I sat down and wept

PART I

Embracing Namibia

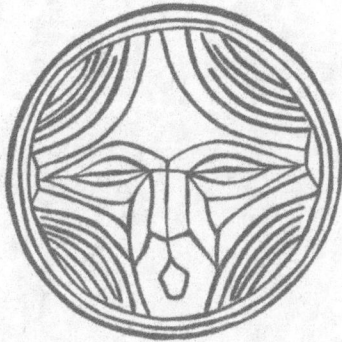

At seven in the morning, the light slants softly across Windhoek and the surrounding hills, before the sun rises high enough to blast its true strength. In the central Mall, traders retrieve their goods from the municipal store – a small locked compound where they can leave things overnight. They come one by one to the sites they have been allocated. A few push supermarket trolleys loaded high with cardboard boxes. Women carry bundles of wrapped cloth on their heads. Two young men struggle with a wooden rhinoceros that is fatter than the pair of them put together. Under the fledgling trees that sprout green only if the rain does come that year, they put out cloths and arrange their goods for sale. Wooden masks with raffia hair and sharp teeth, from the Congo. Green malachite bowls and bracelets from Zambia. Polished, sculptured soapstone figures from Zimbabwe. Brightly beaded necklaces from Kenya. The Namibian products: woven baskets, carved wooden bowls and animals, dolls in the Herero dresses adapted from Western missionaries, wire geckoes, black and white lino-cut prints from budding artists.

Through the traders I walk, to start my day, exchanging greetings with familiar faces, checking for what's new. I skirt round boxes that are being unloaded and head towards the row of shops. At the end is a small bookshop. Reflected in its windows are the crafts from across central and southern Africa that the traders have laid out to sell. Inside are books that reflect the culture and history of the whole continent, with a specific focus on Namibia. I come to the door and unlock it; the air inside is close and slightly dusty. I deposit my briefcase at the back by a desk covered with papers, switch on the computers and then exit once again. I lock up and walk on in search of coffee.

Across the city, soon after five, while it's still dark outside, Doris rises. The house is quiet and everyone else is sleeping. She sits at the kitchen bar and brews her coffee while she contemplates the day ahead. People will be arriving to stay in the small guesthouse she has created at the back of the house. She must prepare rooms for the guests, welcome them, give them whatever they need for their visit, and plan their evening meal. Then she will sit on the phone and sell adverts for the travel guide she publishes with her husband, Clive. In the afternoon she will come to the bookshop to join me. She downs two cups of coffee before her various jobs start, showers, pulls a brush quickly through her chin-length, fair hair, and

1

dresses in loose linen trousers and a long shirt. She puts on gold-rimmed glasses, lights a cigarette and gets going. She won't stop until after it's dark once more and they and their three grown-up children, and any guests, have been fed.

Doris came to Namibia in the mid 1960s, when she was just 16, and South Africa still ruled the country in defiance of international law, imposing apartheid laws to separate black and white, and entrenching white privilege and economic power. She saw the political campaigns against that system and the involvement of the churches on issues of human rights abuses, and she married Clive, a South African journalist sympathetic to change, who was covering political developments in the country.

When we met, we recognised a kindred spirit in each other and we unraveled our stories over glasses of white wine. Doris grew up in Germany, in Frankfurt in the 1950s, while I grew up in Leeds, in the north of England, just two years younger than her. We had many childhood memories that mirrored each other, growing up in the post-war years, although from what she says about shortages and the destruction of Frankfurt, it sounded as if Doris's childhood was much harder than mine.

Her father was captured by the Soviet army at the end of the war and spent five years in a Siberian prison camp (returning a socialist). Her mother had to flee Eastern Germany, where the family had lived, as the barriers between East and West went up, taking Doris's three sisters first and then returning for her furniture and her piano, which she took with her, much later, when they retired to Namibia, or 'South West Africa' as it was then called. Doris was the child born after her father came home from Siberia, her sisters many years older than she was, and forever distant from her.

Deedee is at Eros, the in-town airport for local flights. It's one of the few flat places in a city dominated by hills, with a runway long enough for small aircraft but not big jets. She sits on one of the few chairs in the small departure lounge and sifts through her papers, making notes, waiting for the flight north to Ondangwa to be called; there she will facilitate a workshop on community development projects.

Her knee-length skirt is sand-coloured so it will not show the dust of northern towns; her top a pale blue. Her legs and feet are tanned from canoeing at the coast. She runs her hand through thick brown hair, newly cut, feeling where it is shaped into the neck, and wondering if it's too short.

She checks her watch, packs away her papers and takes out her mobile phone. She sends messages to friends, arranging to get together when she's back in Windhoek; to her son, Timmy (15), to remind him what to take to school; and her daughter, Sarah (13), to wish her well for the day.

Organised, confident, in love with Namibia and with life, Deedee has travelled the world more than most of her American compatriots, both with her parents and on her own from a young age.

She is an inquiring spirit, interested in why people do things and what they believe. As a student, she followed an eclectic combination of comparative religion and economics. Then she met and married Michael, a visiting theology scholar from South Africa.

'I fell in love with his singing,' she says.

They moved to South Africa, and worked in Cape Town and Namaqualand in the early 1980s. After that, they came to Namibia, living in Windhoek and then in Walvis Bay, Namibia's main port. They moved back to Windhoek in 1990, to a house in the black township of Katutura with a large dusty yard next to a small Anglican church, where Michael was the parish priest. They were the only white couple in Katutura.

I met them at the Waterberg, a flat-topped mountain plateau rising on red cliffs above what is already the high plateau of central Namibia. You can hear the sound of water there and the reeds rustle in the breeze. There is always some greenery, even in the dry season. It was the first place I visited that made me understand why people love this land.

At the foot of the Waterberg cliffs is a wildlife resort, with bungalows for visitors to hire. My husband, Peter, our two children, and I went there one weekend and were wrongly booked into the bungalow that Deedee, Michael and their children were already occupying. We introduced ourselves and talked while the accommodation was sorted out.

One of the first things I noticed about Deedee: a white woman with two brown children, just like me. They came through another path – adoption – but it created an extra dimension to the bond between us.

Sandy sees her children, Brigit (16) and Ross (14), off to school, and returns to bed to steal more sleep. Her husband, Ted, drops them and continues to his office. An hour later, Sandy gets up and showers. She squeezes gel onto her hands, runs her fingers through blonde-streaked hair, and crunches the loose curls into a semblance of order. She puts on an ankle-length skirt with a paisley pattern in muted orange and reds, a plain white, thin-strapped, tank top, and picks up a beige jacket. She dons three beaded necklaces and half a dozen bangles on each wrist, and heads off to her theatre in the centre of town.

Sandy first came to Namibia in 1975, on a four-month road trip with an Australian boyfriend, from what was then Rhodesia (now Zimbabwe), through South Africa, Botswana and Namibia. Their small car broke down repeatedly and they eventually abandoned it on the side of the road in the Transkei in South Africa, and hiked back to Rhodesia. She came to stay in Namibia seven years later, by then married to Ted, another Zimbabwean. He had been working with a low-income housing project in Zimbabwe, which was by then independent, and was invited to help establish a similar project in Namibia.

Sandy has lived in and seen the Independence of Zambia, Malawi, Zimbabwe and then Namibia. She has travelled far in other ways as well, from the enclosed white communities in which she grew up to community theatre in Namibia, helping young Namibians to express themselves and their heritage in dramatic form.

When she came to live in Namibia, Sandy worked at first as a shipping clerk, but she lost her job because she spent too much time and energy in children's theatre. Soon after Independence, she set up a 'Theatre in the Park', right in front of the Parliament buildings, for children interested in acting, and to offer space for small, experimental, plays. Unfortunately, the building was soon needed by the government, so Sandy found another venue down the road, in an old building from the German colonial period of the early twentieth century, which she converted into a Theatre School with small stage and tiered seating.

In addition, she puts on full-scale productions at the National Theatre and directed the Namibian performances at the international EXPOs in Lisbon in 1998 and Hannover in 2000 – representations of story, music and dance that picked up traditional forms of self-expression, and melded them into a whole to celebrate Namibia.

4

Big heart. Big hugs. Big hair. Big gestures. Big dreams. Sandy throws herself into each production. Ted quietly supports her through it all. He is straightforward and steady, the rock on which their family rests while Sandy lives through the highs and lows.

Sandy is enthusiastic, outspoken, never bland. She treats everyone the same way, with directness and candour. Most people love her but some don't like the fact that she is so independent, that she will do what she wants and not what others want, that she can make things happen.

Bente is in her garden with a cup of coffee, soaking up the moments of quiet before a hectic day. Then she calls her two girls, Ida (13) and Nora (10), to come and gets the car out of the garage for the school run. She drops them at the International School and drives on across town to the office of the Swedish non-governmental organisation of which she is the representative in Namibia, although she herself is Norwegian.

She is calm and clear, full of compassion, not accepting fools but gentle and firm with everyone. Slim, fit, tanned, with very short, fine, blond, hair, and wire-rimmed glasses, she has a quick response to everything and is always busy. When she's not at work, she adapts the clothes she buys to suit her taste, adding appliquéd African designs, or beads, or seeds, re-knitting two sweaters into a new style of her own, cutting and sewing dresses and jackets.

Bente trained as a teacher in Norway, and then worked in the 1980s for an NGO that supported health and education projects for Namibians in exile in Angola and Zambia, under the care of the liberation movement SWAPO (the South West Africa People's Organisation). In the course of her work, she met Uazuvara, a Namibian activist and film-maker, and an old friend of ours. Eighteen years older than Bente, he had a history of falling in love, and of women falling in love with him, by correspondence, because of the beautiful letters he wrote.

'This is something different, with Bente,' he told us after he introduced her to us,

They came to live in Namibia with the great influx of people returning home at the time of Independence, just like we did. But they did not stay long. A couple of years later, Uazuvara had a serious car accident, suffering head injuries when his car spun off a gravel road and overturned. After the accident, he had to give up his job. He decided he needed a more peaceful life, and he took Bente and the girls back to Norway.

Bente had settled into life in Namibia. She enjoyed her own role as gender officer for the Swedish embassy, working with women's organisations across the country and with Government programmes to address gender issues. She didn't want to leave. But considerations about Uazuvara's health were paramount, so they returned to Arendal, her hometown. Nine years later, she decided they had to come back so their girls could get to know their Namibian heritage. She realised she would have to find a job here and she did. She moved the family once more, to take up a two-year posting in Windhoek with an NGO working to build civil society organisations and a focus on community nutrition and health, and training teachers.

Coming out of the Norwegian solidarity movement, Bente has none of the baggage I have as an Englishwoman, with Britain's colonial past in Africa. I envy her that, and her ability to respond to African issues in a straightforward manner.

Jane starts her day with a cup of tea in bed, brought to her by her husband Helao. He saw her father doing this for her mother and decided that's what husbands do.

'It's not just the tea,' Jane says, running her hand through shoulder-length, dark brown, wavy, hair. 'It's that moment of caring it symbolises. I'm not much good in the morning without it.'

Like Bente, Jane has become the breadwinner, caring for an older husband. He is in his late sixties now, and retired, while she is still in her forties. She does much to help members of his extended family, even though many of them did not care for her when she first arrived.

Jane is sensitive to the lives and stories of others, her empathy fired by a background in drama. She brings this to her work, first with volunteer teachers and now with people with HIV/AIDS. She feels that she doesn't do enough for those in need but I fear her becoming drained by her constant giving. I fear that the day might come when she is the surviving matriarch of the family, providing and caring for many, and perhaps without her husband to support her emotionally.

I knew Jane before we both came to Namibia, through our involvement in solidarity work in England in support of the movements to end apartheid in Namibia and South Africa. She was working for a scholarship agency in London. Peter and I were helping Namibians who had left the country in search of tertiary education not available to black people under the South African occupation. We looked for courses for them in Britain and sent them to Jane for scholarships.

In 1984, in response to international pressure on them to allow Namibia independence, the South African government released a group of 15 Namibian political prisoners who had been imprisoned on Robben Island for their involvement in SWAPO's armed struggle. Helao was one of this group. Some of them went immediately to England, to study. They were given scholarships by the organisation Jane worked for, and that is how Jane and Helao met.

In Namibia, after Independence, Jane and I didn't see much of each other at first. We both avoided too obviously teaming up with other inter-racial couples, and I was in awe of Helao and other former political prisoners like him. He had spent 18 years in South African jails. What do you say to someone who has endured so much? I feel that Helao is a being of a different order. He has an utter gentleness with people, combined with clear, firm convictions, which I have only glimpsed elsewhere in other political prisoners and some religious leaders.

I am also in awe of Jane herself; her commitment to community and her kindness make me feel frivolous in comparison. Her name should have been Ruth: *'And your people shall be my people.'* But Jane laughs out loud at the thought of being seen as respectable and responsible, and one of my joys is getting to know her better.

Tricia braces herself for school; it's not the children she despairs of but her own conditions of employment. She has many times the experience of her young, international colleagues, but this is not appreciated by the school and she resents the fact that she has been hired on a much lower, local salary.

Tricia taught my children when they were small, encouraging and honouring them the way a true teacher should. She is a warm, outgoing person, with a self-deprecating sense of humour, and a real love of children. Short, with dark brown hair, a few streaks of grey showing, and a ready, dimpled smile.

Tricia has lived and worked most of her adult life in different African countries and retains a Scot's sense of anti-imperialism. She and her husband Richard spent many years in Zambia. She taught in local schools while Richard worked in a distance-learning unit for Namibians in exile, with a particular focus on the learning of English.

They loved Zambia, and came to identify with the Namibians with whom they worked, and their cause of liberation. When they moved to Namibia at Independence and made it their home, however, Tricia began to feel isolated. Her children were away at school in Britain; the Namibians she had counted as friends in Lusaka became Government Ministers, or their wives, and she saw them rarely.

Then there was the dry, hard spirit of white Windhoek that made her stomach knot and gave her nausea. Looking for teaching jobs soon after she arrived, she found herself wedged into the tight, disciplinarian structures of the education system inherited from the days of South African rule. She eventually moved to the newly formed International School, set up by Namibian parents whose children had started school outside the country, and who wanted them to continue to learn in a more creative environment than that offered by local schools. The principals and senior teachers came from outside the country and did not recognise her knowledge of Namibian history and people; nor did they fully utilise her skills and enthusiasm.

Tricia feels that she is getting nowhere. She resents how engrossed Richard is in his work, developing materials for the distance education unit at the University of Namibia. She begins to feel her age.

'In another ten years I will retire and have nothing financially to show for my years of teaching, nothing I can call my own,' she says.

Isobel organises her mornings to allow for coffee with her husband Hugo after he has dropped the children, Jan Barend (15) and Kara (12) at school. By eight o'clock they have already had 30 minutes together at the Brasilian café in the centre of town. It is away from domestic surroundings, a time to talk about each other and the day ahead, their expectations and concerns, before going their separate ways. Hugo moves on to his architectural practice. Isobel has a freer programme since she gave up her job as a top legal drafter in the Office of the Attorney General two years before.

Isobel is quick and quirky, with a lawyer's eye for detail. She notices what people say and do, picking up on things that others miss in a story in the newspaper, observing behaviour others overlook in social interactions. She brings little pieces of information from different sources into conversations – people she has spoken to and things she's read.

Isobel grew up in South Africa, in Potchefstroom and Port Elizabeth, but she strains against her Afrikaner heritage. She and Hugo chose to leave South Africa in 1985 because of the state of emergency and the police repression of political activity: they did not want to be part of it. They had heard about an opening in an architectural firm in Windhoek, through friends they had made while backpacking in Europe. Hugo applied and got the job.

'Coming to Namibia was like a breath of fresh air,' he says. 'The relations between people in Namibia were so much better than in South Africa.'

They have made Namibia their home. But Isobel feels that her South African family does not understand her commitment to her adopted country, especially since the Independence of Namibia brought the black majority to power four years before this happened in South Africa, while many white South Africans were still resisting change.

Law is in Isobel's blood. Both her parents are also lawyers. Her father is a well known South African lawyer. Her mother started to train at the age of 40 and thirty years later, she is still practising.

Isobel herself chose to be a lawyer as she left school, studied and then practised for twenty years, until she decided that it was time to take a break and develop other areas of her life; so she gave up her job at the age of 45.

'I didn't want to forever be doing what I chose to do when I was 17,' she explains. 'I wanted to develop my creativity and allow my intuition to come to the fore.'

She enrolled in an LLM degree in international trade law and took up art. She keeps all options open for her future.

'I am waiting to see what I will be when I grow up,' she says.

The Brasilian café lies in a walkway just off Windhoek's busy central arcade, with its long-established cafés that are the early morning haunt of businessmen and MPs. These cafés offer strong, filtered German coffee and fried-egg breakfasts or brotchen – crispy white bread rolls made German style – filled with meat or cheese or egg. The Brasilian is different; it's the first dedicated coffee shop with cappuccinos, lattes, decaf, Italian-style sandwiches, muffins, croissants and fruit salad openers to the day.

Large, glass-panelled doors fold open in the summer, but there are no other windows, so the interior is dark, giving it the feel of a bar. Flags from different countries hang from the ceiling like pennants, and mugs from all corners of the world are lined up on a shelf around the wall. A television shows aerobics or sport – cricket, football and rugby. Behind the counter are dozens of different types of coffee beans. The smell of coffee being ground draws in customers from the walkway outside. The hiss of the machines, as espressos and cappuccinos are made, intersperses conversations.

Friday mornings, at 7.30, after all our children have been dropped at school, six of us meet at the Brasilian for coffee: Deedee, Sandy, Bente, Jane, Isobel and I. Tricia has already started her first lesson. Doris is busy providing breakfast for her guests.

Isobel and Hugo started this ritual. It was their idea to have coffee together before going to their respective offices. It was hard for them to stay on their own, though. In a small community, there is always someone you know at the next table.

Deedee joined them first, when she became the local project liaison officer for an American foundation, whose office was nearby. Then Sandy. Then they drew me in, and later the other Jane, and Bente when she returned to Windhoek. So, on Fridays, if Hugo is there, he leaves or moves to join another table, giving us time together. Everyone knows that is where we will be at 7.30 on Fridays – until 8.00 or 8.30 or even 9.00 if we have no urgent meetings. We extend our time together as we uncover more we want to talk about and share.

Deedee is the convener of the group, the glue that keeps us together. She is the one who sends us messages to make sure we will be there on Friday, and see if any of us needs a lift.

She or Isobel are the first to arrive, racing to get a table before other customers come, so we don't have to sit in a long line along the counter at the side. We ease ourselves onto bar stools round the high hexagonal table with wood surround and blood-red tiled top. We bring our lives to the table.

Isobel draws on past experiences at work, the characters amongst her family and friends, and tales that illustrate the lessons of life. Tall, slim, with short hair streaked in blonde and red, she calls us to order. 'I've got a story for you' she says, and we settle in to listen.

Sandy swings in later with arms open to embrace us.

'Sweethearts! Darlings! How are you, my best, best friends?' she cries, and kisses each of us in turn.

'Hello my darling,' she says, turning to the waitress. 'Skinny cappuccino please.'

'Make that two,' adds Deedee.

'And another,' I say. Jane drinks tea but the rest of us are so consistent with our cappuccino orders that the waitresses bring them as soon as we look in their direction.

'I have to tell you about this idea I've had for a future production,' says Sandy.

'Go on, Sands, tell us about it,' says Deedee.

'Everyman,' Sandy says.

We look confused.

'The mediaeval morality play! It deals with all the important issues.'

'Like what?' asks Isobel.

'How we live our lives and who your friends are!'

'Sounds good,' Jane says. She calls the waitress over and orders more hot water for her tea.

'I have vague memories of it from school,' I say, 'but I wasn't interested at that age.'

'Oh it's gorgeous,' says Sandy. 'The list of characters is amazing. There's Knowledge, Fellowship, Confession, Discretion.'

'It sounds like a list of names in Zimbabwe,' I say.

'Yes!'

'And what happens?' asks Bente.

'God sends Death to Everyman and he doesn't want to go on his own, so he asks his friends to go with him.'

11

'And who does?' asks Deedee.

'Good Deeds.'

'Aahh.'

'So what are you thinking of doing with it?' Jane asks.

'Well, just think of what fun you could have casting those characters, or reflecting topical issues here,' Sandy says.

'It sounds fascinating, Sands,' says Deedee, 'I can't wait to see how you develop the idea.' Then she looks round at the rest of us: 'Let's order something to eat. I'm starving.' She calls the waitress.

'Fruit salad, please,' she tells her. Sandy and Jane order the same. 'What about you?' she asks me.

'I'll have one too,' I say, 'but not too many apples,' I tell the waitress.

Deedee laughs. 'What's wrong with the apples, Jane-Jane?'

'They keep them in the fridge, and they're always cold and hard,' I say, smiling.

I turn to Sandy: 'How are your parents? Have you spoken to them recently?' There's been news of unrest in Zimbabwe, where they live.

'They're doing alright.' Sandy replies. 'Look, it's not easy, but they're living in a small place and they've got friends around them.'

'I read an interesting article about Zimbabwe the other day,' I tell them. 'It said that adoption there is very rare. Apparently people in Zimbabwe don't like to adopt children because they won't know the child's totem.'

'I was given a totem by people I was working with in the north of Namibia,' says Deedee.

'What are you?' We all want to know.

'I'm a Zebra!' she says.

'And I've been given a totem by Helao's family,' adds Jane. She hesitates. 'I'm a Cow!' We laugh out loud.

'I want to tell you about what happened after Uazuvara's father died,' Bente says. 'You know, he was the keeper of the holy fire,' she pauses and takes a sip of her cappuccino.

'When he passed away, the elders had to identify the person in the family who would inherit that responsibility. Since his older brother died, Uazuvara became the eldest living son, and he was worried they would tell him he was inheriting the holy fire. Although it's an honour, it would be difficult for us, because he would have to be at the homestead all the time to keep the fire burning.'

She pauses. 'Now, in the custom of their clan, anyone who has a yellow cow is not eligible to inherit the holy fire... Well, they decided that Uazuvara has a yellow cow – me! So he couldn't inherit!'

We roar with laughter. The people at the table next to us stop talking and look in our direction. We wave at them.

'Sorry!' and continue laughing.

The waitress brings the fruit salad in large white bowls and we shuffle our cups around to make space for them on the table.

'How's the new job going, Jane? I ask. She is heading a programme on HIV/AIDS set up by a Danish non-governmental organisation.

'I'd rather be doing this than working with the volunteers,' she says. 'They were wonderful young people, but I felt so responsible for them, being their main contact here when they were all so far from home. I was forever sorting out problems for them, taking them to the doctor, and so on. It just never ended! But it's humbling getting to know people who have HIV/AIDS and who are trying to live positively.'

'What's the focus of your programme?' Isobel asks.

'To bridge the gap between knowledge and practice and change risk-taking behaviour,' Jane says.

'That's the heart of the matter,' I comment. Educational materials in different languages go to schools, students, teachers, nurses and other professionals, but the HIV/AIDS infection rate is still one of the highest in the world.

'Yes, it's a challenge,' Jane says.

'I have to tell you, I just love my job,' says Deedee. She had set up the children's desk of the Council of Churches in Namibia before Independence and worked in early childhood education for many years, before deciding it was time to move on to broader development work.

'I love being in contact with people on the ground involved in different projects,' she goes on, 'and helping them gain access to possible funding. The only problem is that I have no decision-making power, because our office comes under the regional representative in South Africa.'

'Mmm. I know what you mean, about being connected at local level,' Bente says, nodding her head. 'One of the projects we support is a small farmers' community in the north that builds houses using bottles as bricks, and produces stoves that burn less wood. It's good when it's possible to help people generate local income.'

'One of the most important things, I think, is getting the size right,' I say. 'That's what I've learnt from my bookshop. You read of big projects that won't be sustainable after the donors have gone, or big private investments that you know will never cover their costs. It's not easy finding the right level at which to operate.'

'How's the bookshop going?' Deedee asks.

'Quite well,' I answer, 'but it's a struggle. Not many people buy books.'

'Do you think that's changing?'

'Well, literacy levels are going up and some people have more disposable income,' I say, 'but for most people, books are a luxury they can't afford.'

It's 2002, twelve years after Independence. Windhoek is no longer the small conservative town it was when I first arrived. The streets then were peopled mostly by whites; shops and cafés closed early; the town was deserted at night; and there were physical, political and psychological distances between black and white, and between different ethnic groups.

Now, the town is still quiet at night but not so deserted. Windhoek centre is cosmopolitan, with cafés full of young people of all nationalities and races, including black Namibians who speak the best German in the country, having been schooled in the German Democratic Republic before Independence. Their return forced the previously all-white German schools to open up and face, if not embrace, change.

Economic and political stability has encouraged the development of a black middle class, who have left their previous homes in the township and populated other parts of the city. Residential divides are difficult to change, however. Middle-income and higher-income areas are increasingly integrated but the poor areas are still 99 per cent black. We have the same structural problems as South Africa, the same legacy of racial separation but, because of Namibia's small population – just two million people – we believe it will be easier to overcome.

I arrived in Namibia in December 1989, soon after the first free and fair elections, leaving a quiet life in an American university town, abruptly ended by the pull of Namibian politics. The unexpected coming together of different factors had culminated in South Africa withdrawing to allow the United Nations to pave the way to Independence. By then I had lived Namibia for years. I already referred to the country as 'home'.

My first home was in Leeds, an industrialised textile town in northern England, with buildings blackened by smoke from factories and household fires, and thick yellow smog each November, through which we could not drive or even walk to school. Our house was large and detached, made out of stone, with a very large garden, apple trees, and outbuildings that had once been for horses and carriage. To one side of it were more stone houses and terraces. To the other side, the roads led down towards a tannery that gave off a terrible smell. There were rows of tiny red-brick terrace houses built for workers, which backed up against each other, two small rooms on the ground floor and two on the first floor, no bathrooms, and shared outside toilets in adjoining alleyways.

My first memory is of my father carrying me in the crook of his arm as he walked up the garden path to our house, shortly before we moved there. I was two. The house was empty and neglected when my parents bought it. I remember running through grass in the garden that had not been cut for years and was taller than me, and playing there with my older sister and brother, and later my younger sister as well.

Boys caught stealing apples from our garden were chased back towards the terraces. Coalmen with horse-drawn carts, and faces black with soot, emptied bags of coal down chutes that led into our cellar. Door-to-door salesmen came with brushes and cloths. Frenchmen on bicycles, wearing berets, sold garlic from long bunches slung over their shoulders. Men looking for old clothes or household objects called over the garden hedge to ask us if we had any. I was aware that we lived in the big house; that we had much more than other people around us; and that we spoke with a different accent (my mother comes from the south of England, although my father is a Yorkshireman).

I became aware of the world beyond Britain at the age of ten, during the Cuban missile crisis of 1962, when I heard adults talk about a pending Third World War. The following year, we got a television and one of the first things we saw was the funeral of US President John F.

Kennedy. We were the first generation of British children to learn about the world through TV images: Biafran children starving during the Nigerian civil war of the late 1960s; demonstrations against the Vietnam War; student protests in Paris, London and the USA; 'the troubles' in Northern Ireland when Protestants and Catholics fought each other, and British soldiers were sent in. New organisations committed to helping poorer countries were established. Our church formed a Third World First group, to which I belonged, to raise funds for self-help, educational and health projects in Africa and Asia.

Against this background I sat down, aged 17, to try to choose what I would study at university. I didn't really want to go. I had always wanted to do something in the medical field. At the age of seven, I had wanted to be a surgeon. At eleven, it was a doctor. By 15, it was physiotherapy, which wasn't a university course in those days. However, my mother had been unable to take up a scholarship to study French at university because of the Second World War, and she was determined that her three daughters would not miss the chance. My elder sister, Sarah, sat me down at a table in the bay window looking over the garden and helped me go through the handbook that listed available courses. I agreed to do English Literature but only if there was no Anglo-Saxon component. My first choice was the University of Sussex, and I went there for an interview for a degree in English Literature in the School of African and Asian Studies. I fell in love with the site and the atmosphere, and was offered a place.

At Sussex, I met black and white African students, Asians, and British students who had lived in Africa or Asia. I moved away from my old school friends from Leeds, as I made new ones from around the world. I got to know black Zimbabwean students and found out what life was like under the white minority regime headed by Ian Smith. I became involved in campaigns on Southern Africa. The Sussex Southern Africa Committee invited a speaker to talk about the liberation struggle in Mozambique, led by FRELIMO, and I wanted to find out more. I felt that the issues at stake in Southern Africa were the most important in the world.

I moved away from literature and did an MA in African Politics at Birmingham University, finishing my thesis in London in 1974, while cleaning offices. Then I went to work as a Scholarship Officer for World University Service (WUS), an NGO helping those who were denied

16

education in their own countries. They had programmes for students from southern Africa, and from Chile, where General Pinochet had just overthrown the democratically elected Government of President Allende.

My job entailed going round universities and encouraging students to raise funds to cover the maintenance side of the scholarships – accommodation and food – while appealing to the university management to waive their fees. My focus was on students from southern Africa. There were many Zimbabweans and South Africans in Britain at that time, but almost no Namibians.

WUS wanted to start a Namibia programme and sent me to meet Bishop Colin Winter, an Anglican bishop who had been deported from Namibia by the South African authorities for speaking out against what they were doing in the country. He had opened a Namibia Peace Centre outside Oxford and a small group of Namibians came to stay with him while they studied nearby. Bishop Winter was dedicated to the cause of Namibian freedom. He told me what he was doing and said I should meet the SWAPO Representative for the UK and Western Europe, Peter Katjavivi. A carbon copy of the letter I wrote to introduce myself to Peter was given to me six years later, as a souvenir, when WUS emptied their files of old correspondence. It was the year Peter and I married.

We met for the first time in London in 1975, at a meeting between British NGOs and the liberation movements of Southern Africa. It was convened to look at ways of providing humanitarian assistance to tens of thousands of people from Zimbabwe, Mozambique, Angola, Namibia and South Africa, who were under the care of the liberation movements in centres in Zambia and Tanzania. The representatives of the liberation movements sat at one side of a long oval table. Those of us from the NGOs were seated opposite them.

I was immediately struck by Peter. Thoughtful and clear, he was able to communicate with both sides. He moved his hands as he spoke, putting them together in front of him at times, fingertips and thumbs of his long fingers touching, to emphasise a point he was making. Tall, in a grey corduroy suit with white shirt and blue tie, wearing brown glasses, his hair slightly receding at the brow, a little beard making his oval face look longer.

We met once or twice again and discussed the question of scholarships for Namibians. But my contract with WUS had been for one year only, and at the end of that period, I left. I wanted to move away from the NGO world and do something more political. I prepared publicity materials for an Anti-Apartheid Movement conference on the position of women in South Africa. A few months later, I got a call from Peter's assistant.

'I'm leaving to join the BBC,' she said, and paused. 'Peter wants to know if you're interested in working with him.' I accepted.

Peter had left Namibia in 1962 in search of education and to work with SWAPO for Namibian independence. He was totally dedicated to his work. This kept us late at the office, planning meetings with politicians and NGOs, corresponding with people around the world who were interested in Namibia, and preparing booklets and other publicity materials. He was adept at writing press statements in taxis on the way to the airport, because he travelled so much.

When Peter and I met, we were both with other partners, but we spent much longer together than we did at our respective homes. I threw myself into the work. I was late for personal appointments, missed dinners with friends and went into the office at weekends. My friends all got annoyed with me; my partner Michael did as well. The intensity of Peter's work brought us very close. Gradually, we fell in love. Peter's son Patji (then six), his partner Kirsten's three other children from her former marriage, to whom he had been a father figure, and Kirsten and Michael, paid the price.

After working full-time for SWAPO for 15 years, from 1964 to 1979, Peter resigned his post as Secretary for Information and Publicity and went to study at the University of Warwick. I found a job as Editorial Assistant with *AFRICA Magazine* – a current affairs magazine with a focus on Africa. For the first time, Peter and I were able to spend time together without the stress of his work.

A few months after he started at Warwick, I went to join him there. I commuted each day to London. It was an hour's journey on the train and half an hour to get to the station each morning. The university campus was outside Coventry, in the countryside. Each morning at six, Peter walked me through the woods to get the bus into the station. When I returned in the evening, he had cooked a meal, becoming an expert at chicken roasted in soy sauce, with rice and sweet corn.

After completing his Masters, Peter went on to do his doctorate at Oxford University, researching Namibian nationalism and its international dimensions. We arrived there in the autumn of 1980, six months after the Independence of Zimbabwe, thinking that independence for Namibia could not be far away (it took another ten years). We were allocated a bed-sitting room in an old house right opposite his college. It was a big, high-ceilinged room in an old, Victorian house, overlooking a neglected garden. A tiny kitchenette was partitioned off at one side of the room and there was a narrow bathroom in what was once a corridor.

I continued to commute to London for a year and then found a job as an editor with an academic book publisher in Oxford. I traded my daily train journey for a 20-minute walk along the canal to work, past sandstone colleges that shone with warmth when the sun touched them but looked cold and pale in the shadow of the clouds. Ancient alleyways carried the ghosts of students going back hundreds of years. Bookshops covered every imaginable subject and literature from all over the world. The covered market had bright stalls of clothes, fresh fruit, pheasants and wild deer hanging outside the butchers.

We lived in Oxford for eight years. We scraped to buy our first home – a one-bedroom flat near a large car manufacturing plant – on the basis of my salary and Peter's scholarship. After he had completed his DPhil, Peter became Director of a small NGO we had set up together with other friends. Its mission was to help Namibians coming to Britain to study.

It was in Oxford that we married, in 1981. Three years later, we had our first child, Perivi. My parents travelled down from Leeds the day before Perivi was born, to stay with my grandmother nearby and be ready to come and help us.

'Don't give birth this weekend,' my mother told me. 'Let me finish some things for Granny first.' I didn't follow her instructions, going into labour on Sunday at midday and into the hospital that afternoon. There were complications, as the baby's heartbeat was much too fast during each contraction. They wanted to do an emergency Caesarean and took Peter off to scrub up, but in the end it wasn't necessary. The moment the baby was born, they took it to the side to clear its lungs. On the birthing bed without my glasses, I couldn't clearly see our child.

'How is it? How is it? Is the baby alright?' I asked anxiously.

'It's a boy,' they said.

'How is it?'

'He has ten fingers and ten toes. He looks fine.' They brought him over and gave him to me.

Peter comes from the Herero community and their tradition is to name a child in relation to something said or done around the time of the birth. '*Perivi?*' means 'How is it?' in OtjiHerero. It can refer to a person or to the state of the world. Since I kept asking this question immediately after the birth, this was the name we chose for him.

A few weeks after Perivi was born, Patji's mother Kirsten brought him to see his new brother. She gave me a bottle of red wine.

'It's good for nursing mothers,' Kirsten told me. 'It gives you iron and helps ensure the baby gets a good night's sleep!'

Peter had been visiting Patji in London but this was the first time that Patji (eleven then) had come to visit us.

When Perivi was three, we took him to Botswana to meet members of Peter's family who had driven to Gaborone from Windhoek for that purpose. We stayed with old friends of my sister Sarah's, who were living there, while the Namibian contingent stayed in a bed and breakfast place nearby. Wherever we went, the Batswana greeted us all in turn.

'*Dumela, Ma* – Good morning, Ma'am,' to me.

'*Dumela, Ra* – Good morning, Sir,' to Peter and also to Perivi, according him great respect.

After a day, Perivi decided to respond: 'My name's not "Ra", it's "Perivi".'

Peter's sister, Elisabeth, his cousin, Gerson, and one of Gerson's daughters, Unomuinjo, drove for 12 hours to get from Windhoek to Gaborone. Peter hadn't seen them for 25 years.

The other passenger in the car from Windhoek was Peter's 24-year-old daughter, Uanaingi, whom he had never met. When he left Namibia in 1962, he didn't know his girlfriend was pregnant, and he couldn't easily get news from home when he was based in other African countries in the early 1960s. It was not until he went to London in 1968, to open the first SWAPO office there, that he got news from a visiting Namibian friend who told Peter that he had a daughter (then five years old).

Peter had another older child as well, a son, Kavesorere, born the year before Peter left Namibia.

'Tell me more about Kavesorere.' I said to Peter when he told me about him. 'Where did he grow up?'

'He was born in Windhoek but I saw him only twice. He was taken to the village to be brought up by his grandmother, as often happens. My family stayed in close touch with his mother and grandmother, particularly Gerson, but I left the country 18 months after he was born.'

'Where is he now?'

Peter produced his only photo of his son, sent to him not long before, wearing the uniform of the South West Africa Territorial Force (SWATF), an army of Namibian conscripts formed by the South African regime to fight SWAPO, pitting son, in this case literally, against father.

We had just a few days in Gaborone with the family, my first contact with Peter's relatives other than some nieces and nephews who had come to Britain to study, and Peter's cousin Luther – Gerson's brother. We filled the time with talks and walks and meals kindly hosted by the friends with whom we were staying. It wasn't possible for Peter to catch up on so many years in that short time or get to know Uanaingi well, but it was, nonetheless, a delight for him. Uanaingi, tall like her father, and with his eyes, was shy and didn't talk much, but when she did, she showed the same sense of humour as her father, even though she had not grown up with him.

When they had to leave to drive back to Namibia again, Perivi climbed into their car and got behind the steering wheel.

'I'm going too!' he declared.

The following year, Uanaingi came to stay with us in Oxford. Peter was away, so I went to pick her up at the airport. We enrolled her in the local Further Education College but it was hard for her at first. We bought her warmer clothes, and a friend gave her an ankle-length wool coat, but it took time for her to adjust to the much colder climate. She was still shy; she didn't know either of us, really; and she knew very little English. She had had a poor schooling, in Afrikaans, interrupted by a long period with TB, and a child of her own – a little girl, Diana, one year older than Perivi, who was being looked after by Uanaingi's mother.

I took Uanaingi with me to shops and friends, to pubs and country houses. I proudly introduced this young, black woman, who is a lot taller than me, as 'my daughter'.

A few months after Uanaingi arrived, Peter received a letter out of the blue, inviting him to go to Yale University in the USA for a year, as a Visiting Fellow in the Southern Africa Research Program. By then I was pregnant again but I was excited at the prospect.

We flew to America when I was seven and a half months' pregnant, the last week the airline would take me. We were late leaving Oxford. Peter had a meeting that went on longer than expected. I was putting things up into the loft at the last minute, in my nightgown, pregnant belly resting on the ladder being held by Uanaingi and another Namibian friend. My parents came to collect us and take us via my grandmother, with whom we were supposed to have a leisurely lunch. She had turned 100 the year before. But we had to fly in, say goodbye, and leave ten minutes later, taking smoked salmon sandwiches with us to eat on the way to the airport.

Uanaingi stayed in Oxford, with other Namibian students who were there. She came to visit us in the USA the following year, and talked non-stop with us, in English. She later moved on to Liverpool to do a Business Studies degree.

Yale University is a wealthy, mostly white, university in a poor black town, New Haven. We lived on the border between the two. To the right out of our house was one of the university libraries, at the edge

22

of the university area, and an ice-hockey rink. To the left, the houses became shabbier; the gardens more neglected, and further still it became dangerous. People looked concerned when we told them the name of the street where we lived. In the middle of the night I sometimes heard gunshots.

We rented a narrow, three-storied house, with two rooms on each floor. It was unfurnished except for a vast fridge and dishwashing machine we couldn't use because we didn't have enough crockery. We bought the basics from yard sales and second-hand shops – two beds, a travel cot for the baby to come, a sofa, three chairs, three knives, forks and spoons, a TV and a desk. We had no car, so we walked with Perivi to his day-care centre, to the university or to the shops in town. People began to recognise us – the rare sight of an inter-racial family, and walking at that.

The walking was good for me, and after I went into labour, everything happened very fast. We phoned a visiting South African scholar whom we had asked to stay with Perivi when my time came, and he arrived. A taxi took us to the hospital, the driver calling ahead to give them updates on how frequently my contractions came. The obstetrician got there just in time. Three hours later, we had a beautiful daughter.

'You can make a phone call,' the nurses told me.

'Even overseas?'

'Yes.'

I phoned my parents, reaching them early in the morning, before breakfast, although it was still the middle of the night for us.

'What will you call her?' my mother asked.

'I think she will be Isabel,' I replied, wanting to name her after my farther's mother who died earlier that year. I was holding her in my arms and she made a small sound.

'I can hear her!' my mother called excitedly. 'What does she look like?'

'She looks like a Japanese princess,' I said. Pale skin, straight black hair, and almond eyes, like Uanaingi's.

We had given Perivi an English middle name, John, after my father. We gave Isabel a Herero middle name, Tueumuna, from the phrase *Ouje tueumuna* – we have seen the world.

The shifts in world politics that helped to bring about change in Namibia happened seemingly suddenly. In 1988, before Isabel was born, talks began between the Soviet Union, the USA, South Africa, Cuba, the UN and the Frontline States of Southern Africa, about Namibia and Angola. Throughout the 1980s, the question of Namibia's independence had been hampered by the Republican administration in the USA insisting that there should be a withdrawal of Cuban troops from Angola at the same time as any withdrawal of South African troops from Namibia. These talks addressed this issue for the first time. The opening up of the Soviet Union and the defeat of South African troops at Cuito Cuanavale in Angola in early 1988 helped to make this possible. SWAPO worked with the UN and the Frontline States but were not represented directly in the talks. They were, however, continuously consulted and briefed by the Frontline States.

In December 1988, it was announced that agreement had been reached for the United Nations to go to Namibia and supervise and control the holding of free and fair elections that would lead to Independence. In April 1989, the UN Special Representative for Namibia, Martti Ahtisaari, went to head the UN presence in the country. Seven thousand UN police and soldiers were to go as well. We knew Ahtisaari and we went to New York to see him in his office, high in the UN building, before he left. We wished him the best and said we hoped to see him there soon. Five-year-old Perivi had a serious look on his face.

'When there are only four South African soldiers left, I'm going to Namibia,' he said to Ahtisaari.

As it became clear that the elections were going to go ahead, Peter decided to return to take part in them, as many thousands of other Namibians were doing. He left in July 1989 in a new dark blue suit we bought the week before, with presents packed for family members. I could not imagine what he felt like to be going home after 27 years in exile. I stayed with the children in the USA until we knew that it was safe for us to go as well.

There was hardly any news about Namibia in the American media during the election process. I got phone calls and messages from Peter and information through the Namibian and UN networks, but it was hard to feel it, hard to believe it was going to hold. However, from 9 to 11 November 1989, the elections took place peacefully. Namibians queued for hours in the sun to vote, at the exact same time that East German citizens were pouring over the Berlin Wall and breaking it down.

Six weeks after the elections, not knowing what to expect, I flew from New York to Namibia for the first time with Perivi and Isabel (then just one year old). We had to change in London and had the whole day there, so I visited my brother, John, and his family. We went for a walk in the park; it was damp and cold. Then we returned to the airport. Heat greeted us in Johannesburg, where we had another day's wait until the flight that night to Windhoek. All my anxieties came to the fore, as we landed in apartheid South Africa but Peter was there to meet us. He took us to rest in a hotel near the airport, where the children spent much of the time splashing in the pool.

It was dark when we arrived in Namibia. We made the 40-minute trip from the airport into Windhoek without seeing anything. We passed through open land, with only the occasional dot of light from a distant farmhouse. We stopped in a house to briefly greet Gerson and Luther's mother, Inaa. Peter was very keen that I should meet her straight away but I was overwhelmed. We had come so far, both geographically and politically. I didn't know what to say, and I knew that she didn't speak English.

'Kora? – How are you?' I tried, using one of my few Herero words. 'I'm so pleased to meet you. I'm so pleased to be here. I can't really believe it.' I didn't know how to express the excitement, tiredness, fear, and strangeness that I felt.

We stayed in a borrowed house for my first Christmas in the southern hemisphere. It was the hottest time of year, before the rains. Outside the towns with their watered gardens, the colours were yellow, brown, grey and orange, unlike the greys and greens I knew from Europe and the USA, or other African countries I had visited. The stark branches of thorn trees stood out against bare earth and bright blue sky. Mountains covered in small thorn bushes, with no leaves since the winter, looked grey and uninviting.

We drove to meet Peter's family in Ovitoto, travelling north from Windhoek for 60 km towards the small town of Okahandja and then east for another 35 km on a gravel road that went up and down over rocky hills and across dry, sandy, riverbeds. Dust flew whenever another car passed. Ovitoto was an African reserve, into which one of the Herero communities had been pushed, first by German colonial forces and then, further into the hills, by the South African authorities that had ruled Namibia. The Herero people, pastoral nomads, had traditionally roamed central Namibia with large herds of cattle. In Ovitoto and other similar reserves, they were confined to the poorest land, which was now badly overgrazed. There were few facilities, no electricity, and very poor roads.

We arrived in Okandjira, where Peter grew up with his mother's aunt, Maria, and he showed us the site of the house in which they had lived; it was no longer standing. His aunt had died in 1970, and his mother Uerieta had died in 1983, the year before Perivi was born. After hearing of his mother's death, Peter had closed in on himself for months. He didn't speak about how he felt. He hadn't informed his mother when he went into exile in 1962, to protect her from police harassment. Yet she was harassed later when Peter was one of the leading spokesmen of SWAPO and his name became well-known in Namibia. The police visited and questioned her constantly.

Three of Peter's aunts and an uncle still lived in Okandjira and we went to meet them. They were living in a row of small tin shacks, made out of corrugated iron and old oil drums, beaten flat. Inside each hut, on a cement floor, lay a mattress on a mat, and small piles of belongings at the back. We had taken boxes of tea, sugar, maize meal and bread, and oranges, biscuits and sweets as a Christmas treat for the children. Peter's uncle was terribly thin; his trousers torn. His aunts were wearing Herero dress: cotton, long-sleeved, ankle-length dresses with full skirts and the *otjikaeva* headdress made of cloth wrapped round the top of the head, stretched sideways into points, to represent the horns of the cattle that are so central to Herero culture and society. This has come to be regarded as traditional Herero dress, although it was derived from those introduced by the missionaries in the nineteenth century.

We sat under a small tree, dogs lying beside us, panting in the shade, while Peter talked to his aunts and uncle, they to him, and they to us, through him. Children came to look at us. Perivi and Isabel were listless in the heat. We had small juice boxes in the car but I didn't want to give them any, because we didn't have enough for all the other children. I struggled with the heat as well. My large, heavy, tortoise-shell glasses that had seemed so fashionable in the USA kept slipping down my nose with the sweat.

We drove on further into Ovitoto, through similar villages. Thin cows foraged in small patches of grass amongst the sand. Goats were eating pods that had fallen from the thorn trees. Through the window, I saw the shine of something on the bushes and thought there were raindrops on them. When we stopped, however, I went to look and saw that it was the white of the thorns themselves, 6 centimetres long.

The road got worse and we had to drive over sheer rock to get to Okasuvandjiuo, whose name means 'the place where you can rest'. This was the settlement where Inaa and two of Gerson's brothers lived. We stayed overnight in the house of one of the brother's, Obed. It was another tin house, but larger and stronger. There was one big room, its walls lined inside with hardboard to provide protection against the heat of summer and the cold winter nights. A double bed dominated the room. Obed's sister-in-law had freshly ironed the sheets for us, using an old-fashioned hot-iron into which embers from the wood fire that burned outside were placed to heat it up. A wardrobe stood in one corner; a coffee table and two armchairs at one side. In the corner was a high pile of suitcases.

'What are all the suitcases for?' I asked Peter.

'Storage space,' he replied.

A covered area in the front of the house held basins for washing and kitchen equipment. Cooking was done on the open fire in heavy, three-legged, cast-iron pots, blackened from the smoke. Water had to be carried from a well the other side of the valley. There were no toilets, just a roll of toilet paper and a choice of directions to head in.

In the morning, Perivi went outside in his shorts and started to play with a boy the same age, who showed him how to flip the little goats, pulling up one hind leg and toppling them over in a somersault. In turn, he shared his crayons and paper with his newfound friend. Isabel, in blue cotton dungarees, her dark brown hair a mass of loose curls, bent over the wash basin outside, watching her father shave. She put soap on her face and tried to copy him.

I sat on an old plastic chair under a tree at the side of the fire, trying to come to terms with this environment, harsher than anything I'd ever experienced before, and impressed at the dignity of the people who had found a way of living there. Inaa and her sister Atuto came out of their house and sat on the concrete step near me.

I greeted them: *'Moro Inaa, Moro Atuto, muapenduka?'*

'*Moro muatje* – morning my child,' Atuto said and started to sing a hymn.

In Windhoek, we caught up with old friends from SWAPO, including Sandra and Mosé, whose house in Lusaka had been Peter's home when he visited the SWAPO headquarters there. Mosé was Peter's cousin and close friend; they had grown up together in Ovitoto. His father and Peter's Aunt Maria were active elders in the church and used to sing together. Mosé met his wife, Sandra, an African American from Los Angeles, when he studied in the USA. They had gone to live and work in Lusaka, where Mosé was Head of the Education Department in the United Nations Institute for Namibia, set up to train young Namibians in preparation for independence.

Mosé, like Peter, had been involved in SWAPO's campaign. They were both elected members of the Constituent Assembly, which had the task of drawing up a Constitution for Namibia. They were both on the Constitutional Committee chaired by Hage Geingob that produced the first draft. Sandra had been in Namibia throughout the election process, and could feel the changes that had already taken place. I could still not believe that Independence was coming.

After a three-week stay, the children and I returned to the USA. Peter came with us. Our suitcases did not make it for some days. Our coats were in the cases, so we arrived in the freezing temperatures of New York in early January in the light clothing we had been wearing in Namibia. I was most concerned about Isabel and Perivi, and we bought them new jackets at the airport before boarding the Connecticut Limousine (actually a small bus) to take us to New Haven.

Peter returned to Namibia at the end of January and over the next six weeks, I packed up our belongings and organised our move. Peter was adamant that his family should be repatriated by the UN, as other Namibian families were. I travelled with the children to Washington by train on a freezing cold, wet, day in February, for a meeting with the UN High Commission for Refugees. They did not help us because we had some income in the form of Peter's fellowship, so we bought tickets with Zambian Airways. In mid-March 1990, I flew with Perivi and Isabel from New York to Lusaka, then to Johannesburg and Windhoek. We had five pieces of hand luggage; the biggest was full of Perivi's toys.

Although our life had been dependent on political developments in Southern Africa, I was not ready for Independence when it came. I had settled into life in the USA, and enjoyed the excellent day care facilities for the children, the university seminars on Southern Africa in which I had participated, the people we knew, and the research on South Africa that I had started, working towards a book that had just been accepted for publication.

Coming to Namibia just before Independence, and having missed the election process, I was also out of step with political developments. I was still in the mode of solidarity politics. I believed that the world was divided into those who were on the side of the Namibian people and those who were not. I expected most white Namibians to be racist and reacted adversely to the sound of Afrikaans. But I was behind the times. In the Constitutional Committee and the Constituent Assembly as a whole, elected representatives from across the political divide had sat together to discuss and formulate a constitution, and decisions had been taken by consensus. This process had moved Namibian political life forward in a peaceful and constructive manner. Always open to talking to people from different political persuasions, Peter was able to interact with people we had hitherto labeled as opponents or puppets. I found it more difficult.

I felt this strongly at a reception given by the outgoing South African Administrator General, Louis Pienaar, two days before Independence. It was his farewell, before he moved out of the official residence and handed it over to the incoming President, Sam Nujoma. The reception was held at the residence, a German-era rectangular sandstone building with red corrugated iron roof in the centre of Windhoek, almost opposite the Parliament; palm trees that welcome the visitor to the front of the house; and pink and white-flowering oleander bushes growing through the fence.

The reception was held in the early evening, as the sun went down over the hills of the Khomas Hochland, shining into the terrace on the western side of the residence. Members of the Constituent Assembly, members of the UN Transitional Assistance Group (UNTAG) and foreign observer missions, businessmen and women, and the media were there. Waiters dressed in black trousers and white shirts carried trays of drinks and finger food to serve the guests. I wore a scarlet lacy skirt with matching short-sleeved tunic, given to me by a Namibian friend as we had left the USA. It was the first time I had ever owned or worn a 'cocktail' dress.

There was an air of eager anticipation yet the guests were very relaxed. I saw SWAPO leaders rubbing shoulders with opposition politicians and making jokes with the top brass of the South African Defence Force. I didn't know what to say to them or how to behave. My dream of celebrating Namibian Independence had not included those whom SWAPO had fought against. As time went on, though, I took my lead from the SWAPO Government and accepted the new politics of reconciliation, working with people from different backgrounds and different political persuasions to try to build Namibia.

On 20 March, the eve of Independence, a different celebration was held – an elegant seated dinner for 300 guests, given by the United Nations. We were seated at round tables and served many different courses. High flower displays placed in the centre of each table made it difficult to see the people on the other side. Dizzy Gillespie played for us. A procession of visiting dignitaries arrived with President Nujoma and the SWAPO leadership: Zambian President Kenneth Kaunda and other African Heads of State, European and the USSR Foreign Ministers, and Nelson Mandela; he had been released the month before after 27 years in prison in South Africa.

After dinner, we made our way to the main stadium. A small contingent of the Namibian Defence Force, newly trained by the British, marched round the stadium and came to a stop in front of the main stand. The United Nations Secretary General, Perez de Cuellar, formally pronounced Namibian independence and President Nujoma took the oath of office. The South African President, F. W. de Klerk was there to witness it. At the stroke of midnight, the South African flag was lowered and the new Namibian flag was raised. President Nujoma saluted. An army band played the new Namibian national anthem for the first time. The fireworks began. Heads of State and Government from across the region and beyond, Yasser Arafat and other world political figures, sat side by side behind President Nujoma. We sat in a section for MPs; Perivi came with us and sat on Peter's knee.

We had lived a simple life before coming to Namibia but, in Windhoek, we became part of the new elite in an inherited system with enormous disparities in income and living conditions. Our first house, located in the suburb of Pioneers Park, had an open-plan reception area – sitting room, dining room and bar – that was bigger than the total floor-space of any house we had lived in before. It even had a separate flat. We bought a sofa and chairs, coffee tables, and bar stools from the previous owner and we sent for our boxes from the UK that had been packed away while we were in America. When they arrived, the contents seemed barely worth the cost of the freight: small ornaments of sentimental value, a few saucepans, vases, cloth that I had kept and intended to make into curtains one day. Except for the books and photos, we could have let everything else go.

The house had three bathrooms, a pool, and a garden of stones, citrus trees and desert plants. I tried to introduce hydrangeas into the garden, but they didn't succeed in Namibia's dry climate. The wisteria I put in thrived, its heavy scent reminding me of English summers.

Before the children and I arrived in Namibia, Peter had looked for someone to clean the house and help look after the children. Alexia had worked for one of the UN election officials and was recommended by her departing employer. She spoke English, which was uncommon but essential for us. She helped fight the dust that blew in with the wind, and washed and ironed the clothes. Perivi played with her when he came home from school. Isabel, struggling to adjust to our huge new house, attached to Alexia when Peter and I were out. When we first moved in, she had run from room to room, crying, trying to find her way, and something familiar.

It was difficult for me to negotiate this new role as an employer. I wasn't used to having any help in our home and I was aware of the dreadful way some people treated their domestic workers, including some of the new black elite. Most domestic workers came to work in municipal buses that went from the black township of Katutura to what had been the white suburbs, where returning professional Namibians found houses. The buses did not go up our road, though, so although she came on a bus in the morning, and walked through to our house, I drove Alexia back to her home in Katutura each day at four in the afternoon.

After six months, Alexia came to live with us. At first, she stayed in a small room at the side of the flat, which had been purpose-built for a domestic worker. Then, when her daughter Turimei (one year younger than Perivi) joined her, we converted the double garage for them, put hardboard up behind the door, a carpet on the floor, and furniture inside. It had an entrance outside the main back door, and Isabel began to spend a lot of time there, playing with Turimei.

Uanaingi also came to live with us, when she returned from the UK after completing her degree. She brought her daughter, Diana, from the village where she had been with her grandmother, and put her into a school in Windhoek. They moved into our flat. Even with all these people, though, we still had so much space.

Before coming to Namibia, the nearest I had ever got to the country was Botswana. I imagined Namibia would be similar, but the physical reality was very different. I had to learn about the actual country: the geography, the people, the languages, the climate, the desert, the rocky hills, the dry riverbeds, the old systems and the new possibilities.

Peter's family were friendly towards me but distanced by language and culture. Old aunties spoke Herero and German. His sisters and cousins spoke Herero and Afrikaans. One niece, a young professional woman, was not happy that her uncle had married a white woman. Other nephews and nieces had studied in Britain and I'd come to know them there. I had been close to my aunts and grandmothers in England and I got on well with the older women in Peter's family. When they talked about him marrying a foreigner, they quoted an old Herero saying:

'*Nokokure kuno'ueenu* – Even in far-away places you will find your own kind.'

Gerson gave me a Herero name, Tuauana, meaning 'we are together'. I started to learn Herero and practised phrases with Peter, Alexia and the aunties, and on the children.

'*Moro, uapenduka?* – Morning, how are you this morning?'

'*Movanga okupuena*? – Would you like a hot drink?'

'*Hama naua* – Sit up.'

I promised myself I would learn Herero before Afrikaans but I began to learn Afrikaans by default, in the post office, the bank and from the switchboard of the Ministry of Education.

I moved from an English language environment into one where English was a rarity, except in official political life and amongst those who had been out of the country to study, or in the liberation movement.

English was chosen as the official language at Independence, to help break Namibia's isolation from the world. It was introduced as the medium of instruction in schools from the fourth grade. Ten African languages were also recognised for use in schools, plus German and Afrikaans. Namibians frequently moved between three or four different languages in the course of a conversation.

It took time to get used to the strong gender roles and social division between men and women. I had already witnessed this in Oxford when young male Namibian students came to visit us. If Peter, rather than I, got up to make them cups of tea, they would be surprised, because this was a task usually performed by women in Namibia. Most Herero men expected their wives to do everything in the home, and to serve them food when they returned from work, even though those wives were almost all working outside the home as well. Most men from other African communities were the same. Children were looked after by women almost exclusively.

Peter was not nearly so chauvinistic but at social gatherings he would gravitate towards the men, while women often grouped together in another area. I was used to us being together in a mixed group of men and women, frequently discussing politics. But I realised that in Namibia I couldn't attach myself to the men if the other women weren't there, so I learned to join the women.

At Independence, the Constituent Assembly was transformed into the National Assembly and its members, including Peter, became Members of Parliament. Mosé was chosen as the first Speaker of the National Assembly. They were both extremely busy and, throughout our first five years in Namibia, I saw little of Peter. He had meetings in the day, the evening and on weekends, and calls through the night from people around the world, phoning to find out how things were going.

Windhoek had changed so much since Peter left that he no longer knew it well. So it was Doris who showed me round and gave me practical advice about settling in. She helped me find a school for Perivi when a promised place at another school fell through – it was hard to find school places because some 40,000 Namibians had returned in the months before Independence. It was Doris who drove me when I had to take Isabel to the Catholic hospital for an ear operation when she was only one year old, and Peter was away. She recommended a doctor, dentist, pharmacist, and showed me where to get the best vegetables that came up by truck from Cape Town on a Thursday. In those days it was carrots, onions and cabbages, not the wide range of vegetables that now fills the supermarket shelves. She told me we could order meat directly from the farm and they would deliver it. So we spent occasional Friday evenings in my kitchen, with a bottle of white wine, cutting meat into chops, steaks and joints for roasting, bagging and labelling them, for the freezer.

We celebrated New Year's Eve at the coast, in Swakopmund, with Doris and her family, setting off fireworks on the road outside their holiday house in a German tradition that had been brought to Namibia. She took us to the Windhoek Show, an annual event at the end of September that had originally been an agricultural show. Year by year, it became more interesting to those of us who were not farmers. Stalls of clothes from Cape Town and further afield were set up. Household gadgets, paintings, woven Namibian carpets, were on display. There was face painting for the children, roundabouts, a Ferris wheel, bumper cars, and fast, spinning rides for teenagers. When our feet were sore, we went to the food area, ordered a cold Windhoek lager and a hot dog made with boerewors – local farmers' sausage. Doris also took us to Independence Avenue in the centre of Windhoek, renamed from the 'Kaiser Strasse' it had been until 1990, and we watched the floats of

WIKA – the Windhoek Karnival – go by. It was another tradition that had come from Germany.

Tricia also helped us with regard to Perivi's schooling. She briefly taught him in his second year at school, while his regular teacher was on maternity leave. I confided in her that I was concerned about the attitude of teachers at the school.

'We thought Perivi's teacher looked so sweet and kind, but we've discovered that she smacks the children,' I said. 'Short, sharp, smacks on the hand, with a ruler.'

'It doesn't surprise me. They're dreadful here,' Tricia confirmed.

'One of the older teachers told Perivi the other day to "beware of the devil" on his shoulder!' I went on. 'They're so hard on these little ones. Perivi's an enthusiastic, playful, seven-year-old, but they're squashing him. I'm wondering whether to move him to the International School.'

'I should, if I were you,' Tricia advised me, and we took her advice. Not long after, she moved there as well. Two years later, Isabel started at the International School, and Tricia taught her in Grades 1 and 2.

Sandy directed Perivi and Isabel at different times in their first plays. At age eleven Isabel was goddess of the birds in a production of 'Children of the Sun'. She wore a golden tunic and a headband round her curls, and moved her arms gracefully as wings – she was doing ballet at the time.

'I don't know if I want to do this,' she said to me early on in the rehearsals. 'I don't like standing up and everyone looking at me.' Sandy helped her overcome her shyness and perform.

Perivi took the role of Edmund in 'The Lion, the Witch and the Wardrobe', at the National Theatre of Namibia, when he was 12.

'It's by far the best role in the play,' Sandy told me. 'It's Edmund who is conflicted, who grows and changes, and finds redemption. The others are just sweet children.'

Deedee drew my family into activities we wouldn't otherwise have undertaken. One year, she suggested a combined family trip canoeing down the Orange River that forms Namibia's southern border with South Africa. I agreed. Peter was not so keen. He learnt to swim late in life, in Oxford, in his forties and he doesn't like water much.

The 'canoes' were rubber rafts provided by the company who organised the trip. They arranged the food and cooked for us each night. We had to each take light clothing, a swimming costume, towel and sleeping bag, and pack those into waterproofing that was stowed in the raft. There were four rafts, six or eight people to each. One of the organisers came in each raft, and everyone helped with the paddling. We had to negotiate little rapids where there were rocks underneath, and steer the rafts through them at the best place, but there were times when the river was wide, the waters smooth and we let the current take us.

Isabel and Deedee's daughter Sarah (both seven) were good paddlers. I paddled on and off; Peter sat rather nervously and paddled occasionally. We all wore life jackets. When we got too hot, we took them off and let ourselves drop backwards into the water. We swam for a while, hauled ourselves back into the raft and let the sun dry our clothes on us; the evaporation cooled us down. It was just after Christmas and very hot. One afternoon we moored at the bank under large trees. The children and I spent two hours sitting in the water, in the shade, to escape the heat. Peter was on the bank. I climbed out of the water to see him.

'Wow! It's like walking into an oven,' I said.

'I reckon it must be 45 degrees,' said one of the organisers.

The information provided in advance about the trip had recommended that, to avoid sunburn, we should wear long-sleeved shirts and long shorts to cover our knees. Deedee and I complied. Most other people wore shorts and T-shirts. There were three young women lawyers from Cape Town who wore black bikinis almost all the time.

I had on baggy culottes, a shirt with a collar and a huge straw hat that covered my face, neck and shoulders.

'I think we're rather overdressed!' I laughed to Deedee. 'Like two Edwardian ladies boating in England!' She laughed in agreement.

I put factor 30 suntan lotion on myself, and factor 15 on the children but it was Peter who got burnt; he was wearing shorts and by the end of the second day his thighs were burnt from being exposed to the sun all that time.

The other people on the trip looked at the eight of us as if they couldn't quite work us out.

'What do they think of us, Deedee?' I asked. 'Here we are: two white women, one black man, four brown children.'

'And Michael!' Deedee laughed. 'Where do they think the priest fits in?'

'He's blessing us!' I replied, laughing with her.

In the absence of my English family, and Peter's absences due to work, these new friends became very important to me. It was also important for me to find something to do, other than being at home with the children. In the USA, I had been working on a book on South Africa, and I set up a small study in our house in Windhoek and tried to continue with it. I had brought documents and books with me from America, in anticipation of not finding many in Windhoek. I was right.

'The worst desert in Namibia is the book desert,' I told friends and family in England.

It was hard to concentrate on South Africa while everyone around me was finding ways of contributing to the birth of Namibia, full of possibilities, and finding new ways of doing things at all levels of society. It was also hard to sit quietly on my own and write when other people were busy. I wanted to be part of things.

'What can I do?' I asked Peter.

'There's lots of things you can do,' he said. 'What would interest you most?'

'You know I've always dreamed of publishing in Namibia one day,' I replied. 'I wonder if it would be possible.'

I spoke to politicians, printers and journalists about it.

'The market's too small,' they all said. 'You can't make it work.'

'There's no such word as "can't",' my primary teacher had always said.

I was brought up to believe that I could make things happen if I wanted to, and I was excited by the stories to be told about Namibia. So six months after I had arrived, I took a leap of faith and set up my own publishing company. I wanted to call it 'Namibian Publishing House', like the Zimbabwe Publishing House that friends of ours had set up soon after the Independence of Zimbabwe. They were interested in publishing in Namibia as well, and I agreed to become their agent.

'That name is taken,' I was told at the Register of Companies.

'By whom?'

'Gamsberg'. It was the only publishing company in Namibia at the time. Set up before Independence, it had published books in German and Afrikaans and the African languages of Namibia, under the education system introduced by South Africa, which had different curricula for the different communities. They had registered the name 'Namibia Publishing House' but hadn't used it.

After long consideration and playing around with different names, I settled on 'New Namibia Books'. My stated aims were 'to build peace, justice and unity and publish new books for the new education system'.

I sat on the terrace of a local hotel with visitors from a British company, Heinemann, who published for Africa and also published African writing. As we drank tea, we discussed how I might work with them. I agreed to be their agent and they gave me some business advice.

'Keep an eye on your cash flow,' they said and showed me how to draw up a chart with anticipated income and expenditure.

I had no business plan, no financial or sales experience and no capital to start with, but Heinemann gave me an advance against commission on the expected sales of some highly regarded secondary-school science textbooks they had published for Lesotho.

'We don't want African science,' was the comment of the Under Secretary for formal education and chair of the science panel (an Afrikaner), when these books were assessed one year after Independence.

So New Namibia Books started to develop a course of science textbooks for Namibia, which we co-published with Heinemann, who provided editorial guidance and support and financed the design and printing. We brought in Namibian teachers as authors, and members of a newly established upgrading programme for science and maths teachers. We met for six months at four in the afternoon, twice a week, for editorial sessions with them that continued into the evening.

The first book I published was a Life Skills book for junior secondary school that had already been approved for use in schools when its author came to me with the manuscript. She had worked as a Guidance teacher under the old education system. There were sections in it on study methods, relationships, banking, and others concerning protocol, how to lay tables and how to address people.

As the science textbooks were developed, approved and bought in schools, I was able to employ three people to assist me. I began to publish the books I dreamt of. *Song of the Namib*, an illustrated poem for children about the song of the wind in the Namib desert. Five children's stories that had been developed at a Build a Book Workshop in which I participated, with Sandy as well. She dramatised one of the stories I published and directed a performance of it at the launch of the books the following year.

I published traditional tales, Namibian fiction and life stories – especially by women – history books, books on democracy, the standing rules and procedures of the National Assembly (working with the Speaker, our old friend Mosé). I funded some of them from income from sales of the science books; others were assisted by non-governmental organisations active in the cultural field. Our two bestsellers were *The Price of Freedom*, a personal memoir written by a woman who had walked across the Namibia–Angola border at the age of 12 to go into exile, and *Last Steps to Uhuru*, a social history of the last two years before Independence and the first two years afterwards.

I also helped set up a book publishers' association in Namibia that held discussions with the Ministry of Education about textbook provision, and organised book displays; and a book development council that brought together writers, printers, publishers, booksellers and librarians. It held book festivals in different regions of the country, to try to develop a love of reading. I was on the Board of the African Publishers' Network (APNET), set up in 1992, which supports indigenous publishing across the continent.

The bookshop came five years after I started publishing, when it became clear that New Namibia Books needed an outlet to sell our books directly to the public. I remember the scepticism that greeted me.

'Namibians don't read,' I was told by those in the book trade who survived by selling textbooks to schools.

'Only the Germans read,' was another comment. But I believed that it would work if books of interest could be brought to people, and we opened at a site in the centre of town where there was a busy throng of people walking past.

I chose to sell books that were not otherwise available – books on African culture, history, politics, literature, Namibian writings and books about Namibia. It worked. Young men snatched up titles on the Black American activist, Malcolm X, and Kwame Nkrumah – the first President of Ghana and one of the fathers of Pan-Africanism. Tourists bought the Namibian flora and fauna books. Academics came for history titles, the classics of African literature, developmental books and those on the environment and women's rights. Some leading members of Government and society came in to buy, and sometimes even the Prime Minister, Hage Geingob, would come into the bookshop on a Saturday morning to see what we had, his security officer a few paces behind.

Two years after Independence, the President, Sam Nujoma, appointed Peter as Special Adviser on Higher Education. A National Commission examined current and anticipated demand for higher education, the human resource requirements of the country, and questions of feasibility. It was decided that a former Academy, set up under South African rule, be transformed into the first national university.

The Academy had provided limited academic training for black students, while whites had had access to universities in South Africa, some of which were recognised as world-class, but which were distorted by South Africa's policies and philosophy of racial separation.

The President appointed Peter as the first Vice-Chancellor of the university, and it was formally established on the day of my 40th birthday.

'Lucky you, Jane!' Sandy told me at a small party we had at home later that day to celebrate my birthday. 'Peter's given you a *fabulous present*. He's given you a whole university!'

Peter brought in a group of advisers to work with him as a Transitional Planning Team, and develop the new systems. They were all black men – academics from Africa and the Caribbean. Some white staff members from the old Academy, who were taken up into the university, did not like this at all and would not cooperate. As time went on, Peter brought in academics from Europe and America as well as Africa.

Peter oversaw the university's growth and development, the opening of new faculties for law and agriculture, centres for human rights, justice training and distance education, and a language centre for the upgrading of English language skills. Medicine and engineering faculties were too costly to set up at that stage.

Along the way, he encountered enormous resistance to change. When the university moved into an extensive complex that had previously been a whites-only teacher training college and had only ever had a few hundred students, the bathrooms were vandalised by some departing staff members. There were battles over curricula and new decision-making structures. There was opposition from a few white lawyers to the establishment of the Law Faculty, saying that it was not necessary because there were already enough lawyers in the country (most of them white). However, people gradually accepted the change and the university has since flourished.

This year, 2002, we celebrate ten years since its establishment. At the Graduation Day we sit in a packed hall at one of the local hotels. Huge displays of flowers decorate the corridors and the platform in the hall, where the top academics sit – the Deans of Faculties and members of the University Senate and Council, made up of academics, community leaders and businessmen and women. The Chancellor (President Nujoma) and the Vice-Chancellor (Peter), sit on two wooden chairs in the centre of the front row of the platform, wearing ceremonial black academic robes designed specifically for the university. The Chancellor's robe has a thick gold-coloured band round the neck and down the front. The Vice-Chancellor's is similar, but silver. Both wear academic mortarboards with tassles, as do the academics on the platform and in the hall. Different coloured stoles draped over the shoulders indicate different faculties.

Diplomats and Government Ministers occupy the first rows in the body of the hall. I get a privileged seat with them on the front row. On the other side of the aisle sits the academic staff, and then the graduands, wearing black academic gowns that they must return at the end of the day, after having their official photographs taken.

The formal protocol of the occasion demands that once in, people are not allowed to leave, and the ceremony takes up to six hours. I get up very early, have a light breakfast, and avoid having a lot to drink. I put on a vest and a trouser suit, and carry a warm shawl. Although it's April and still quite hot, the air conditioning in the hall is chilling over that length of time.

The Vice-Chancellor, the Chancellor and a Visiting Speaker all give speeches, reflecting the achievements of the university over the year, and addressing issues relevant to higher education, and the development needs of the country. Then the parade of students being awarded their degrees gets under way. Department after department, they queue at the side of the hall. Each student in turn climbs the steps onto the stage, hands over the paper with his/her name on it, and walks across to receive the stole from the Registrar, who places it carefully over head and shoulders. The student's name is read out loud. If they are getting a degree, they are then capped by the Chancellor – the President. Then they descend from the stage and collect their certificates from a table at the side. The students dress up in smart suits or dresses, the women in high heels. They move as slowly as possible across the stage in order to draw out their moment of triumph. Friends block the way as they bustle to take photos of each other.

At this year's ceremony, Isobel is awarded her LLM degree, which she embarked on two years before. Her mother has come from South Africa for the graduation. I stand up to hug Isobel as she comes down from the platform, certificate in hand, cap on head, stole over her shoulders.

'Can you imagine,' she tells the others at the Brasilian later that week, 'I walked across the stage, was capped by the President, came down the steps and there was Jane standing up to greet me, with my mother watching from the back of the hall, because we came late. The aisles were full of grandmothers in traditional skirts waving their fly-whisks, ululating for their children – the first ones in so many families to go to university. To be part of that celebration of achievement. What a moment!'

Isobel recently returned from a visit to her father in South Africa, to sort out his belongings so that he can move into a retirement home. He has had to leave the house where she and her siblings had grew up – their family home – in which he stayed after her mother left years before. Now two of the six children – Isobel and one of her brothers – help him to choose what little it is possible to take with him, and throw away or give away everything else.

'We had to make decisions about family furniture – who could get what or would want what – but also about old clothes, old documents and confidential papers belonging to my father,' she says.

'In the end,' she goes on, 'we threw away a lot, filling a skip that was parked outside the house for that very purpose. Then we thought we had thrown away too much. We put things in the skip, then took them out, then put some back in again, When we left, having finished everything, I looked at the broken chairs and the old rugs lying there, the documents blowing in the wind, wondering about them being made public in this way. It's sad but no one else in the family was prepared to undertake this task, although they started to argue with us later about what they should have been given and what should not have been thrown away.'

As they sorted and packed, Isobel's brother developed a story about the family, their attitudes to their father and to the removal process.

'My brother said we were like a dysfunctional cricket team, with several players unavailable for selection or suspended!'

We laugh but it makes the rest of us think about our parents. All of them are far away and in their seventies and eighties now. Sandy's parents are the nearest, in Zimbabwe. Jane's father is in his nineties, and lives with her sister in England. My parents are also in England; Deedee's in the USA; Bente's in Norway. We talk about how to help them when the time comes, and what we would do if or when our parents die. One day we will have to face our own mortality too, of course, but we don't talk about that.

While in South Africa, Isobel found a photo of her wedding at her father's house. It is her favourite wedding photo – better, she says, than the ones she has at her own home. She brought it back to Windhoek with her and she shows it to us. It's a classic wedding photo – the bride in white, the groom at her side, smiling at the camera, in pretty surroundings.

'Look,' Sandy comments. 'Look at Hugo. See how he has that special smile of his that he has when he's got what he wanted.'

The photo starts a trend, and we all demand to see each other's wedding photos. Jane brings hers the next Friday – a studio photograph of her and Helao.

'Tuli likes to say that she is in the photo too,' says Jane, 'because I was pregnant when we married. There was no one else there except Tuli, our two witnesses and us.' Tuli is Jane's 15-year-old daughter. Her son, Freddie, is 11.

'What about your parents?' we want to know.

'I didn't want them there,' Jane responds. 'They came to know and love Helao but they weren't keen on the marriage at first, and I didn't want any negative feelings around.

In my case, my father quizzed Peter for a long time on their first meeting, asking about his political beliefs, his contribution to the liberation struggle, whether he had been engaged in the armed struggle (he had not), and his visions for the future. He wanted to know whether Namibia had any chance of getting its independence.

By that time, I had already told my parents that Peter and I wanted to get married. He was far from the English professional my parents must have assumed I would choose, and they had no idea of what the future might hold for us.

'It's the children I worry about,' my mother said. 'Will they be accepted?'

'They'll be loved by both sides of the family,' I asserted. I would not defend my choice or try to encourage them to accept Peter. I simply informed them of what we were doing.

When Peter and I got married, I sent invitations to all my aunts and uncles, willing them to come and show that they too accepted my choice, and they did, including my grandmother who was in her nineties and a great-uncle in his eighties.

We married in the Oxford registry office – a small room above a shopping centre, situated almost so that you could do your weekend shopping on the way out. Think of Oxford with all its beautiful buildings and famous spires, and that was what the council put aside for non-religious weddings! We went by taxi into the car park and upstairs in the lift, walked along a narrow corridor, brick-lined on one side and open on the other, into the ante-room of the registry office. We were a party of 15 and there was only just room for us all as we waited.

The couple before us and their witnesses and guests came out of the room where the ceremony was held and we all went in. There was a table at one side of the room, with flowers on it and the book – the registry – that we would sign, and four rows of chairs for the wedding party. I wore a long, muted green and beige, African dress with emerald and white embroidery round the neck and down to the waist at the front. Peter was in a dark three-piece suit. Our vows were short and to the point:

'I call upon these people here present to witness that I, Rosemary Jane Coles, take you, Peter Hitjitevi Katjavivi, to be my lawful wedded husband.'

Peter's cousin Luther came over from Germany to be best man. He and my father signed the registry as our witnesses.

Luther had arrived to stay with us two days before, and another Namibian friend, Frieda, came up from London to be with us as well. The night before the wedding, Peter became quieter and quieter. Luther talked to him while Frieda twisted his hair into tiny plaits, to help him relax (he undid them before going to bed).

We booked a restaurant near our flat for the reception – 40 or so of us, friends and my family. One of my uncles sat opposite a group of Namibian and Ghanaian friends and joked that he felt he was facing the West Indian cricket team. Luther didn't like speaking in public, and didn't want to speak at the reception. We left that to one of the Ghanaians, who entertained us all, making due reference to the Stevie Wonder/Paul McCartney song 'Ebony and Ivory'.

Uazuvara, one of Peter's oldest friends, was also invited to the wedding, but he didn't make it. He had already been married and separated and said he didn't believe in marriage any longer. It took Bente to show him there could be something more to it.

After showing us her wedding photograph, Jane talks about Helao and his comrades. These are the men who launched the armed struggle for independence in 1966, over 30 years ago. They were captured in Namibia, taken to Pretoria (in South Africa), and tortured there. These are the men for whom the notorious Terrorism Act of South Africa was brought into being – enacted in 1967 to deal retrospectively with Namibian freedom fighters who had been arrested the year before. Men who gave up a large part of their adult lives in prison on Robben Island.

'When they were released in the mid-1980s,' Jane tells us, 'they were welcomed into exile by the SWAPO leadership but there was no specific support for them. When they returned home at Independence, there was still no support. They asked the Government for help but were told that they couldn't be given special assistance as other groups would ask for the same. So they took on the task of supporting each other, and they agreed to go to each other's funerals. At the first funeral, one of them turned up without shoes.

'The younger group of Robben Island prisoners, those who were arrested in the mid-1970s, did not have quite the same problems,' she continues. 'They had better education and were more able to get jobs afterwards. A few in Helao's group got into Government, but many had to struggle to survive. Some of those who had no family home were resettled, irony of ironies, into a former South African Defence Force camp with partly derelict buildings and land.'

Helao himself worked in the public service but was forced to retire the moment he turned 60, despite his lifetime service to the country and the fact that some others managed to stay on beyond that age. He had made the mistake of asking the party leaders if he could marry this Englishwoman. They said no, but he went ahead and did so, and they sidelined him thereafter. Jane didn't know about this until he finally told her after they had been married for ten years.

Jane and I have sometimes been mistaken for each other – two English women with the same name married to Namibian men. But our husbands are linked in another way.

'When Peter was sent by Sam Nujoma to the UK in 1968 to open up a SWAPO office there,' I tell her, 'one of his main tasks was to raise funds for the defence of the SWAPO Terrorism Trialists, including Helao.' Jane is intrigued – she had not known.

'We have documents in Peter's boxes,' I say. 'I should dig some out for you to look at. Old leaflets. Appeals to European organisations for support. Information sent out to publicise the case. The President sent Peter with £50 to open up an office in London for this purpose. He went via Cairo where he was given a raincoat by the SWAPO representative there. Then he went to East Germany to get leaflets printed about the plight of the Trialists, while he was waiting for his visa to the UK. There he was given a typewriter to help his work in London. So he arrived in London with £50, a raincoat, a typewriter and the leaflets, and somewhere in a box at the back of the garage we still have the accounts book in which he recorded his first expenditure!'

We never get to the other wedding photographs. I know nothing about Deedee's wedding except that she has told us she played tennis with her brother two hours beforehand and that she and Michael left for South Africa soon afterwards. I know little about Sandy and Ted's wedding except that their reception was held at Leopard Rock Hotel, high up in the Bvumba Mountains in eastern Zimbabwe. Peter and I went there once with friends. We could see far across the border into Mozambique. Some say that on a clear day you can see the Indian Ocean.

If Bente had brought her wedding photos, the others would have seen that Peter was Uazuvara's best man. I couldn't be at the wedding, but I've seen the photos of Bente in her lilac dress. I've heard the stories of Peter's speech, talking about past times he had spent with Uazuvara, extolling his virtues and then commenting on how stubborn Uazuvara is, and telling Bente she must give him a good kick now and then.

At Friday breakfasts with my friends, we move between our personal stories, discussions about work, and the political context of our lives. They are all interwoven. We are touched by what happens in our families and in government, by the changing face of national and regional politics, and Namibia's recent involvement in the war in the Democratic Republic of the Congo (DRC).

At the request of Congolese President Laurent Kabila, troops from Angola, Zimbabwe and Namibia moved into western Congo in 1998/9 to help crush an armed uprising that started in the east of the country. Initially their task was to safeguard the capital Kinshasa and the corridor west to the sea. That much I could understand, but then they moved east towards the Great Lakes, far beyond any place I could think it was in our interests to defend.

After that came a crisis in Caprivi, the long finger of Namibia that reaches into central Africa and a border point where Namibia, Botswana, Zambia and Zimbabwe meet. It's one of Africa's bizarre colonial inheritances, granted to Germany in a deal with the UK in the nineteenth century as a corridor so they could move from German South-West Africa to their East African territories. They had hoped to travel down the Zambezi River but they couldn't get far because of the Victoria Falls.

The Caprivi proved to be a useful launch pad for SWAPO's guerrillas to come into Namibia in the 1960s and begin their armed struggle against South African rule. Later, it became a heavily fortified base for South African troops fighting against SWAPO, and in recent years it has become an apparent focal point for the disaffected from all the countries that surround it. In 1999, Caprivian separatists attacked a military base, airport and radio station in Katima Mulilo, right at the eastern border of Caprivi, killing 13 people. They were met with strong action by the security forces who detained many; hundreds more left the country. Namibia had lost its innocence.

One of the younger former Robben Island prisoners, Ben Ulenga, came out in public that year, condemning government policies and breaking away from SWAPO to form a new political party, the Congress of Democrats. This former fighter, trade union organiser and poet, gave up his ambassadorial post because he objected to the move to allow the Founding President, Sam Nujoma, a third term in office. He was also motivated by his opposition to government policies on the poor, on unemployed former freedom fighters, and on Namibia's military involvement in the DRC.

Ulenga was heavily criticised by SWAPO members and the party press and accused of betraying the liberation struggle. Nevertheless, he was elected as an MP later that year, along with 6 other COD MPs (out of the National Assembly total of 72 MPs). They had almost ten per cent of the vote, higher than any other opposition party, and were set to become the Official Opposition until two other opposition parties hastily agreed to a joint platform. Together, this new coalition had more MPs than COD, so they became the Official Opposition.

The Congress of Democrats has, however, been constrained by differing interests of the people who joined – from those who were dissatisfied with the Government, to young white businessmen looking for a political home, and young black professionals who thought they were not advancing fast enough in the new dispensation.

While our soldiers were in the DRC, Sandy put on a production of the Greek classic 'Lysistrata' at the National Theatre. The title of the play means 'she who disbands armies'. It tells the story of an uprising of women in ancient Athens in opposition to war: they decide to withhold sex from their husbands until the war is over and peace is secured. Sandy worked with young people who had mostly never acted before, building up their skills and their performance, creating an impressive production with a Namibian feel, singers and set, and pointed references to Namibia and the DRC. We all went to see it.

'I think it was Sandy's best ever,' Deedee said at the time, sipping her skinny cappuccino at breakfast at the Brasilian.

'I agree!' said Jane.

'Thanks guys,' Sandy responded.

'You say that about each of Sandy's productions, Deedee!' I pointed out. We laughed.

The Namibian troops began to withdraw from the DRC in 2001. Then, at the beginning of 2002, Jonas Savimbi, the leader of the Angolan rebel movement, UNITA, was killed by government forces. The civil war in Angola, which had raged since Independence in 1975, abruptly ended.

Peace in Southern Angola, UNITA's stronghold, brings peace to north-east Namibia as well. Groups of UNITA soldiers, often with no money or provisions, have been raiding villages on the Namibian side of the border for five years. This now comes to an end.

Angolans start coming over the border with money to spend, providing a welcome boost to local trade. They reach my bookshop as well, and I come to the table one Friday with good business news to share.

'We're doing a booming trade in English/Portuguese dictionaries,' I tell everyone. 'I'm selling 30 at a time. I can't re-order them fast enough. I was speaking to the pharmacist the other day. He says he's selling out of all sorts of things too, even toothpaste, to Angolan customers. And my brother-in-law tells me that you can't get hold of any building materials in Windhoek at the moment because they've been bought out by Angolans who are trucking them across the border to rebuild towns and villages.'

One of our new bookshop customers from Angola is a Dutch man who has been working for years for a non-governmental organisation in Luanda. We start to talk about the situation there, the civil war that was funded by income from oil for the ruling MPLA government, and income from sales of diamonds and ivory for UNITA, and the generals on both sides who profited from those sales.

This is the sort of bookshop work I love – talking to someone with interesting experience, with whom I can share information, views and books. I was always less keen on the administrative detail – the cashing up, book-keeping, checking stock.

When I first opened the bookshop in 1995, I moved a competent administrative assistant from our publishing office to manage the day-to-day business of the shop. I concentrated on keeping up to date with new titles, ordering, sales to libraries, and on our publishing work. The new bookshop manager, insufficiently supervised by me, siphoned off cash over a two-year period before I found out. She was late giving me sales figures, or producing records for the accountant. I tried to get the accounts up to date, but there was always something missing.

'From my experience, when there is this sort of delay, something is wrong,' the young woman auditor told me, looking at me as if she thought I was old enough to have known this.

I took boxes of invoices, cash slips and till records home from the shop and started to try to make sense of them. It was a soulless task, demanding many starts at four in the morning, pouring over the accounts spread across our dining room table.

'Get someone in to do it for you!' Deedee kept saying to me. But I was stubborn and convinced that a book-keeper or accountant would only come back to me with queries, so I might as well try to sort it out myself. In the end, I identified N$25,000 missing (over US$5000 at the time), suspended the bookshop manager, and went through a labour tribunal to state my case against her. She confessed to having taken money out of the till when her relatives came to her in need. I dismissed her. She signed an acknowledgement of guilt and agreed to pay back a certain amount each month but she stopped doing so after a few months and, despite my efforts, the courts seemed helpless in enforcing the agreement.

It was always a struggle to make the bookshop work in such a small market. As long as I was publishing as well, the two sides of the business complemented each other. But New Namibia Books suffered from what so many small independent publishers suffer from – a lack of capital and capacity. I started out with a loan guaranteed against our house and once it was paid off I had no desire to take that risk again.

After nine years, I thought I had built up a viable publishing company with good editorial and production staff and a trainee marketing coordinator who was based in the bookshop, but then it started to unravel. I had increasingly to deal with the administration and financial management rather than the work that I loved best – the actual book development – and while I spent my time sorting out the bookshop accounts, my colleagues made their own decisions about their futures. First, the editor went to study in New York at graduate level, then the publisher and editorial assistant left to work with the new political party, COD. Our production manager emigrated to Canada, and later still the marketing coordinator left to sell cigarettes – a much more lucrative proposition for him. I was loath to make the commitment to training and building up a new team, so in 2000 I accepted an offer from the largest local publisher, Gamsberg, and sold our publishing list to them. At least it would keep our books alive and in print, I rationalised, and focused on trying to keep the bookshop going on its own.

It was after I had been defrauded, and the bookshop manager dismissed, that Doris joined me. She brought new life and laughter to the shop. Together we beefed up the stock, the range of titles and the re-ordering processes, reaching out to school and other libraries, thereby increasing sales.

Doris shares my love of books and my belief that literature contains life's great truths. We sit with Peter and Clive for hours, talking about books we are reading; and about politics, past and present.

Although peace has come to Angola, political conflict in Zimbabwe continues to intensify. The elections in early 2002 are marred by accusations of intimidation and vote rigging. To avoid being expelled because of this, Zimbabwe has withdrawn from the Commonwealth. The economy is suffering; real wages are declining; there is serious labour unrest; a shortage of maize; and the currency is fast losing its value. The expropriation of former white farms has disrupted the production and sale of tobacco, which earns much of the country's foreign exchange. The land issue has also provoked an international outcry, especially in Britain, with its many family ties to whites in Zimbabwe. Britain seems to have forgotten that it promised in the Zimbabwean Independence settlement of 1979 that it would assist financially with land reform.

My first encounter with Zimbabwe was as a child in Leeds, when a new girl came to join my school. She was my first real friend, someone else to play with other than my brother and sisters and the boys next door. Joy was different from the other girls – suntanned, freckled and tomboyish, with an accent that fascinated me. We rode our bikes together up and down the road, with pieces of cardboard pegged to the spokes of the back wheels so that they would sound like motorbikes. She came from Rhodesia and she talked to me about her life there; the colours of the bush, the animals and how quiet elephants can be as they walk. Joy's family didn't stay long, however; they moved on to Australia and New Zealand and finally settled in South Africa. We kept in touch by letter for some years but then lost contact. As I became involved in the anti-apartheid movement, I feared that she might be on the other side of the political divide.

After I came to Namibia, I thought about Joy from time to time and wondered if I could find her. Fortuitously, my parents gave me a book about her great-grandfather, the explorer Trader Horn, and I eventually wrote to the publisher asking about her whereabouts. Within 24 hours, Joy had contacted me by email, asking me if I was the Jane with whom she had dressed up as characters from *Little Women*.

'It was like opening a window into my childhood,' I tell Deedee, Sandy and Isobel, as we sit on our balcony having tea one afternoon. Tricia is also with us as school has finished.

'I remember dressing up a lot but I had forgotten that we re-enacted *Little Women*. It brought back so many memories. I dug out an old hardback copy of the book and have just finished reading it. I rediscovered Jo, the tomboy sister, who wanted to write, and with whom I always identified. And guess what? Jo ended up marrying a foreign professor who was older than her. I thought of Peter and me and wondered, is this is how we determine our future at a young age?'

My next encounter with Zimbabweans was as a student at Sussex. I began to follow the movement towards majority rule. When the Lancaster House Agreement was signed in 1979 and Robert Mugabe won the elections, Peter and I celebrated with champagne in what was then his student accommodation at Warwick University.

Peter and I went to Zimbabwe in 1982, just two years after its Independence. We visited friends in Harare who were in the Government, and those who were not. Two old friends, David and Phyllis, whose publishing company in Harare I later represented, took us to see Great Zimbabwe in the south of the country – the ruins of an eleventh-century African civilisation linked through trade in gold to the East African coast. High, circular, dry-stone walls encircle a 22 metre conical tower at the centre of the ruins. The stones are pale grey, all the same size, small, like bricks, and carved to fit perfectly on top of each other; there's no trace of mortar in between. Little is known about the settlement but it's estimated that up to 25,000 people lived there at its peak.

We walk round the ruins and through the narrow corridors between the walls. Climbing up a rocky outcrop nearby, we come to a temple complex where the stone birds that have become the national symbol of Zimbabwe were found.

For Peter, this was a particularly significant journey. It was 20 years after he had left Namibia, in 1962, to go into exile. He had been 21 then; I was 10.

Peter had traveled east from Windhoek, with two friends, Ferdinand and Brian, crossed into Botswana (then the British Protectorate of Bechuanaland), and north to what was then Southern Rhodesia. They were heading for Dar es Salaam, where SWAPO had its headquarters. In Plumtree, in the south of Rhodesia, they were arrested and imprisoned for three weeks, because they had no papers.

'We were thirsty and we made the mistake of going to a farmer's house nearby to ask for water,' Peter told me when I asked him about the journey.

'The farmer came and asked us where we were from. We said "Bulawayo" but when he asked us where in Bulawayo, he wasn't impressed with our answers. We didn't know any words in Sindebele, so we weren't convincing. He didn't say anything to us but he went and called the police. They came and took us off to jail. I felt really bad, wondering what my mother would think. One of my friends, Ferdinand, regretted having left Namibia and said he just wanted to go home and marry my sister.'

They were taken to court and, while they were waiting to appear, they were approached by an activist of the Zimbabwe African People's Union (ZAPU), one of the liberation movements campaigning for majority rule in Rhodesia. He asked them who they were and they told him. He alerted SWAPO headquarters, who contacted the United Nations. The UN, in turn, requested the British Government (then the colonial power in Southern Rhodesia) to be on the lookout for three young men from South West Africa.

The Rhodesian authorities in the meantime took steps to deport Peter and his friends to South Africa. They were handcuffed, chained at the ankle, and put on a train from Plumtree through Bechuanaland, with a three-guard escort. At Francistown, an Englishman boarded the train, checked their identity, and told them there was a change of plan and they would be stopping in Gaborone. When they got to Gaborone, British officials boarded the train and came to Peter and his friends. They instructed the guards to remove their handcuffs and chains and ordered them off the train and into two cars. Peter and his friends were in one; the guards were in the other. They were taken to the office of a senior British official, who read out their names.

'These three young men are no longer under custody,' he declared. 'They are free. We, the British Government, will assist them in their journey to East Africa.'

'It was the first time I'd heard the word "custody",' Peter told me.

In Zimbabwe in 1982, 20 years after this journey, we wanted to retrace Peter's steps and go by train through Plumtree to Botswana, where he was going to do research amongst the Herero community. These people are the descendants of Hereros who crossed into Botswana as they fled German colonial forces during the uprising against German rule in Namibia in 1904-08. Peter was doing research for his doctorate by then. He wanted to interview elders in the Herero community in

Botswana to learn more about the uprising and about their role in getting Namibia's case heard at the United Nations in the late 1940s.

In Harare, we tried to book a sleeper cabin on a train south to Gaborone but the young black clerk at the train station refused to sell us tickets.

'It's a South African train,' he said, 'going to Johannesburg. You two can't stay together on a South African train. It's not allowed.'

Despite our protestations that Zimbabwe and Botswana were independent and that we had no intention of going into South Africa, and despite producing a copy of our marriage certificate (which I carried because my passport was still in my maiden name), he would not relent. Inter-racial relationships were illegal in South Africa.

We went instead by bus to Bulawayo, overnighted there in a small hotel and found a much more helpful ticket clerk the next day, who sold us tickets for the train to Gaborone. We bought mangoes from a vendor at the station and ate them on the train, getting sticky hands and faces in the process. It was a sleeper cabin and we settled down for the night but I hardly slept. I was afraid that we would sleep through the stop in Gaborone and end up being taken into South Africa, where Peter would have been arrested for his work with SWAPO.

I have visited Zimbabwe many times since then, and tell my friends in Windhoek that I love the place.

'Why?' they want to know.

'Because it's green.' (There are many large trees in contrast to Namibia's small thorn bushes.) 'It's black.' (The accountants and lawyers and managers I meet are black, not white, as they still so often are in Windhoek.) 'And I can speak English to everyone.'

My own work has taken me regularly to Zimbabwe, networking with publishers and with others in the book world there, and participating in meetings of the African Publishers Network (APNET). The annual Zimbabwe International Book Fair (ZIBF), originally started by David and Phyllis in 1983, has been a favourite of mine.

Now the biggest book fair in sub-Saharan Africa, ZIBF is held in Harare's sculpture gardens, with huge stone sculptures offsetting the bookstalls and the art gallery at the side. It is a celebration of African culture and writing. Hundreds of stalls exhibit books published across the continent and books published outside about Africa and/or by

African authors. Writers, publishers, printers, and booksellers come to the book fair. Government ministers from around the continent, dressed in tailored African outfits, flowing robes or bright shirts, share forums addressing education, culture, sustainable publishing and the development of African literature. It is one of the big annual meeting points for people in the book world.

I have missed the past two book fairs because of other commitments, so I'm excited to be going again this year (2002). However, I'm shocked by the changes I see. The book fair is a reduced version of what it used to be, with fewer exhibits; many people I expect to see are absent. The value of the Zimbabwe dollar has dropped drastically, although there is a flourishing parallel market where people exchange foreign currency at many times the official rate. It costs thousands of Zimbabwe dollars to get a taxi from the airport into town, although the price in Namibian Dollars/Rands has not changed. There are many more people selling goods in the streets or hanging around on corners than there used to be and I'm advised not to hail a taxi in the street as I used to, because there have been cases of people being mugged.

I select books from different stands as presents for everyone at home: Peter, Perivi, Isabel and my friends. At the Brasilian, when I get back, I give the others their presents.

'Ooh, new books,' Deedee exclaims. 'Thank you, sweetie.'

'Excellent!' says Sandy and flips through hers eagerly.

I share with them my impressions of my visit.

'The prices of things in the shops are unbelievably high. There are food shortages. People told me that the country is surviving on remittances from Zimbabweans working overseas. They talked about political repression. They said that South Africa could cut the supply of electricity to force political change, and I heard bitter accusations against South African President Mbeki because he doesn't do that. Of course, the international press is full of the expropriation of white farms, but what I found hardest were the stories of political intimidation and the youth militias set up by the government, that train young people before they are allowed to go on to further education, and turn them against their own people.'

Our own President stands firmly behind President Mugabe of Zimbabwe. There are those in the Cabinet who disagree but we do not hear their voices.

Sandy's parents were born in what is now Zimbabwe. They moved to different parts of the old Federation of Rhodesia and Nyasaland but came back to live in Zimbabwe. They come to visit Sandy often. Last year, Sandy's mother celebrated her 70th birthday in Windhoek. We treated her to our birthday breakfast routine, got the waitresses at the Brasilian to lay the table smartly, and organised flowers and sparkling wine. Recovering from cancer, she survives miraculously on half a kidney; but she loved every moment of the breakfast.

Born of British parents in what is now Zimbabwe, Sandy's parents have lived all their lives in different parts of the former Federation of Rhodesia and Nyasaland, staying and teaching in Zimbabwe. Now, a little more than 20 years after Independence, it has been decreed that anyone eligible for another citizenship must choose between that and Zimbabwean citizenship. They apply for and get British citizenship. They are still Zimbabwean residents, but they've lost their right to vote.

Sandy herself, as she applied for Namibian citizenship soon after Independence, had not wanted to relinquish her Zimbabwean connections, but in those days many of us who had come to live in Namibia decided to become citizens. When I made that choice, I described it as like deciding to get married: I wanted to say 'we' instead of 'they'. I wanted to join this new country in the making, where all things seemed possible.

After a peripatetic life with Peter, moving from house to house in England and the USA, settling down in Namibia has been important to me. After we moved into our house in Pioneers Park, I had no intention of moving again. It was from this house that Perivi, and later Isabel, started school. They went to swimming lessons at the municipal pool with a German teacher recommended by Doris, then practised at home in the pool at the back of our house. Isabel learnt to ride a bicycle, pedalling with determination up the slight incline of the road outside. She began to play the piano and take ballet classes too.

These were the years when Perivi played with Doris's youngest son, Ben, who was just two months older than him. Isabel tagged along, climbing trees and wrestling with them, trying to keep up with the boys.

To get to the nearest shops, we walked through an area of veld along a small riverbed that ran between our road and the next. Further through the veld was a sports club where Perivi had karate classes, beside drooping pepper trees that made me sneeze when I took him there. It was in the riverbed that Perivi made his first movie, with a home video camera. He developed the story and organised his friends into acting different roles. I held the camera and was told what to film, but we had no equipment to edit it, so the story remained a jumbled mixture of out-of-sequence scenes.

Family and friends from outside Namibia, including my parents, visited us there and we took them round the country. Luther and Brigitte, his German wife, came, and sometimes Luther on his own, making our home in Namibia his base as well. One Christmas Luther brought his 20-year-old daughter Miriam. Born in East Germany when Luther was studying, she grew up there with her mother Gisela, after Luther moved to West Germany. Miriam's pale, oval face is framed by thick black hair, pulled back into a permanent pony tail; she has her father's dark brown eyes. She met him for the first time since she was tiny after the Berlin Wall came down and she could travel to the West to see him.

Patji also came that same Christmas and turned 18 while he was with us. His name means 'dawn'. It comes from a phrase used by people in the liberation movement: 'Patji ngarikutuke – Let the dawn of freedom come'.

When we lived in England still, Peter went to visit Patji in London but since we had left for the USA and then for Namibia, they hadn't seen much of each other. This was an opportunity for them to have time together. It was the first time Patji had spent more than a weekend with the children and me and I welcomed the chance for us to get to know each other better. I wanted him to feel at home with us but I felt awkward about showing physical affection to Peter in Patji's presence; I didn't want to seem to be claiming him.

Perivi and Isabel loved having Patji, and he was good with them. He got on well with Miriam as well; they were close in age and had much in common, even though they hadn't met before. We took them to the Etosha National Park, and stayed in self-catering bungalows overlooking the waterhole. Patji and Miriam sat up half the night to watch the animals coming to drink. After Etosha, we went to the coast to show them Swakopmund and the desert. Back in Windhoek, we celebrated Patji's 18th birthday quietly at home: a family gathering with his Namibian aunts and uncles, and us, a special meal and champagne.

After six years in Pioneers Park, I started to feel restless. In a city surrounded by hills, with houses balancing on rocks in precarious places, we lived in the only flat part of town. Isabel wanted stairs to slide down; I wanted a view. I mentioned to an estate agent friend that I might be interested in moving and that afternoon she took Perivi and me round three houses, just for fun. We fell in love with the third, in a suburb called Ludwigsdorf on the outskirts of town.

I phoned Peter, insisting on talking to him although he was in the middle of a meeting, and told him that I had found the house I would live in until I died and that he must come and see it. He arrived within half an hour and later that afternoon we fetched Isabel from her ballet class and brought her too. We all loved it. Peter, the children and I went round the house, planning how to use each room, marveling at the mountain that rose up unfenced from the bottom of the garden, directly in front of the house, reminding us of the rocky hills of Ovitoto.

We moved in 1996, in the coldest winter I had ever experienced in Namibia, not realising we would be in the shadow of the mountain from four in the afternoon. It was icy. Huge windows that opened onto the balcony let in the cold; there were no curtains and no heaters, just a wood-fire hearth with a blocked chimney that forced smoke from any fire back into the room. My younger sister, Helen, visiting Africa for the first time, could not believe how cold it was. She borrowed a woolly hat to sleep in, and wore her leather jacket all day, except when the sun came into the front garden and we could bask there, lizard-like, to warm our blood.

Uazuvara and Bente and their girls visited us that winter as well, and four-year-old Nora commented:

'This is a funny place where you have to go outside to get warm.'

The children brought their blankets into the sitting room in the evenings and wrapped themselves up while they were watching television. We wore socks and vests under our pyjamas and piled duvets and blankets over us at night.

Along the width of the house, opposite the mountain, runs a balcony, over two metres deep. It is our favourite feature. We sit on the balcony at the end of the day and watch the sun go down on the Auas Mountains to the south of Windhoek, turning them orange and then purple. We sit and talk with visiting family and friends, sharing tea and ginger biscuits in the afternoon, a glass of wine at the end of the day. Occasionally we have a meal there but the balcony is laid with uneven stone and it's difficult to get a table to balance.

We watch the face and nature of our mountain change with the season, from the sudden burst of green after the first rains, to the bright yellow flowers low on the ground when the rain continues; the dry yellow and grey of winter, and the creamy blossom softening the thorn bushes in August, heralding our short spring. We see eagles soaring above and klipspringers on the rocks. We climb up the mountain past a cave that was inhabited by leopards 20 years ago. From the top we can see the whole city and the hills of the Khomas Hochland stretching away to the west.

The location of our house has brought its problems as the children have grown older, though. It's right at the edge of a city without public transport and we have to take Perivi and Isabel to and from school each day, and take Isabel to and from her afternoon sports and dance classes as well. I can't travel for my own work, when Peter is away, without making elaborate arrangements for Perivi and Isabel. I can't concentrate at work in the afternoon because I get phone calls asking me to bring home milk, bread, chocolates and videos.

Over my love for our home are also laid the night-time worries about how and when Perivi (now a teenager) is coming home at the weekend. I lie awake at night waiting for his footfall past our bedroom window, anxious about his safety in the city at night, where fights and stabbings are all too common.

Perivi leaves the house saying he is going '*kostora* – to the shops', even at eleven o'clock at night, when the shops are long shut. He walks down the steep hill, up the next, and down again, to get to the road where he can find one of the small taxis that drive round Windhoek looking for customers. They take in as many people as they can and drop them off one by one so no one knows how long their journey will take. He meets up with his friends at one of the few clubs in town, or goes to parties in friends' houses. There is one cinema in Windhoek, one swimming pool, one place to play mini-golf, a few squares with basketball hoops. Otherwise there's nothing for teenagers to do. At weekends, he comes home in the middle of the night, at three or four o'clock, walking back up the hills, past barking dogs and private security guards outside some houses, who are all too ready to jump. We get angry with him for staying out so late, but to no avail.

Our home has also been touched by the stresses of my work. For years, the garage has been full of the books I published, samples from the publishers I represent, and filing cabinets full of papers from my business. I feel swamped by it. I've tried for 12 years to encourage writers, to publish and sell their books, and to build a love of reading in Namibia. In addition, I manage the household and look after Perivi and Isabel. It has become too much. My head feels packed with the pressure of all the things I'm trying to juggle and control. I get up feeling tired. I work slowly and without enthusiasm.

After finishing school, Patji studied medicine in London. He came to stay with us in Ludwigsdorf during his housemanship years and worked at the hospital in Katutura. He cycled ten kilometres from the house to the hospital each day, and ten kilometres back up the hills again. He encountered medical conditions he wouldn't have seen in London – late stage tumours and other advanced diseases in patients who hadn't gone to the hospital until they were very ill, and injuries caused by stabbings and fights at the weekend or the month-end, when people got paid and drank too much.

When he completed his studies, Patji came back and worked at Onandjokwe hospital in the north of Namibia. By then he had already decided to specialise in obstetrics/gynaecology. He was immediately put to work helping with Caesarean births and delivering mothers, some of whom who were HIV-positive.

While he was there, he met and fell in love with a young Finnish woman, Heidi. She was visiting the nearby Finnish Lutheran mission centre of Olukonda, where old thatched buildings from the late nineteenth century are kept as a museum. Patji and Heidi spent a year together at Onandjokwe. When we visited them there, they showed us round. The hospital, also built by the Finnish Missionary Society, had its own sauna, in spite of the very hot temperatures outside. When they left to return to London, Heidi was pregnant.

We go to Finland now, for Patji and Heidi's wedding in the small town, Kuortane, where Heidi's father is pastor. We fly to Helsinki from London, overnight there and walk round the city in shirtsleeves and T-shirts because the weather is warm. The next day we travel by train to Kuortane, and are picked up by Patji in an old station wagon. He and Heidi drove over from Norway, where they're living and working. He has Norwegian citizenship because his mother is Norwegian and he found he could finish his specialisation training more quickly there than in England, where they wouldn't recognise the experience he had gained working at Onandjokwe.

The temperature drops sharply the night before the wedding and it's cold inside the church. Heidi wears a classic, sleeveless, cream wedding dress with a pink trim and shawl; Patji wears a dark suit. Heidi's father Kyösti performs the ceremony. Patji and Heidi's 18-month-old son, Egil, is held in turn by Heidi's mother, Kaija and Patji's mother Kirsten.

The reception follows in the hall of a church complex. Small wood chalets are available for guests to stay, right by the lake. Silver birch trees grow in and around the buildings.

Peter sits at the top table with Kirsten and Heidi's parents, Heidi, Patji and Egil. I sit at a long table with Isabel, Perivi, Luther's daughter Miriam, her fiancé Matthias, and some of Patji's friends from his university years in London. One has come over from Brazil. Heidi's aunts and uncles, her sister and three brothers, are there, and Patji's other brother, Muhindo and sister Maya, with their spouses and children. His eldest sister, Beni, is stuck in London because of a strike by airline staff and isn't able to get over for the wedding. I talk about Namibia to Maja, whom I haven't seen for a decade; when we passed through London at times over the years and visited Kirsten, Maja was doing research in the USA.

In the drawing room after the meal, different family members stand up to recite a poem, sing a song, or play some music at the piano. Peter makes a short speech and so does Kirsten. Egil accompanies each pianist, reaching up to touch the keys at one end of the keyboard while they play.

As the older people turn in for the night, the young ones gather at the sauna by the lake. The party continues into the night for them, the brave ones going into the sauna and then throwing themselves into the icy waters afterwards. They get to bed near dawn, not long before the older generation rise for breakfast and continue talking in the dining room.

Returning to Windhoek after the wedding, refreshed and rested, I am surprised by an overwhelming desire to give up the bookshop. It has been a balancing act to keep it going after I sold the publishing list. Most of our sales are to tourists and foreigners based in Namibia. There are Namibians who come as well, but not as many of the educated elite as I had hoped for. My heart is suddenly no longer in it.

The international educational publishers we represent pay us commission on the sale of their titles in Namibia. I thought we could boost sales of these books, increase the commission income and enable the bookshop to continue. But the publishers have asked for more marketing visits to schools and, when our marketing coordinator left, I chose to cut costs by not replacing him. That left the marketing to me.

I know I don't want to make this extra effort, nor continue to sort out the accounts, reconcile the bank statements, check all the figures. I want to step away from it all. Yet this poses all sorts of problems. Who will promote the books we are representing? Who will sell the books I love? Who will employ the people I work with?

One Saturday morning, when Doris and I are both in the bookshop, I take advantage of a quiet period when there are no customers, to tell her how I feel.

'I don't know if I'm going to keep going with the bookshop, Doris. I feel burned out. I dream about finding a nice quiet place and writing, not having to be responsible for all this anymore.'

She looks at me and lights a cigarette. 'They say you have to be very disciplined to write,' she says and pauses.

'I'd be sad if you closed the bookshop, it's been a lifesaver for me. With the kids to look after once again, and Clive, and the guidebook and everything, I was getting really depressed. I went to see the doctor before I started working with you here. He suggested anti-depressants but I didn't want to take them. Then you asked me to join you and I didn't feel I needed them.'

I knew that Clive had closed in on himself after leaving his job as a journalist to go into public relations, which he didn't like. It had made their family life difficult at times. But I didn't realise that Doris had been depressed as well. Two of their children had returned to the family home after being away at school and university, and had partners who were constantly present. So Doris has had to look after seven people, as well as their bed and breakfast guests, work on the guidebook she and Clive publish every year, and in the bookshop in the afternoons.

Despite the way I feel, I tell myself that I should stay on to make the books we stock available to Namibia, because most are not found in other bookshops; to continue to provide jobs to the people I employ; to provide an escape for Doris. So I soldier on.

Instead of changing things at work, I decide we need to move, and despite my initial intention of living in our house forever, I start to look at other houses. No one else in the family thinks we need to move, but I forge ahead. I find a little cottage with a thatched roof and huge eucalyptus tree at the side, at the bottom of the garden of another house. The dry grassy smell of the thatch seduces me. There's a tiny garden and a tiny pool with dark blue ceramic tiles, just outside the sitting room. I imagine myself returning from work, making a cup of tea and sitting outside with my feet in the pool to cool off. I imagine walking to the small shopping centre around the corner. I imagine Isabel (now 13) walking to her new school, Perivi (18) coming and going independently from the room at the rear of the house with its own external door. He has just left school and started a course in media and communications at the University of Namibia. I imagine the loosening of demands on my time and attention. This is what captivates me most of all.

On a second visit to the house I take Doris with me.

'No,' she says. "It's sweet, but it's too small. The bedroom that would be Isabel's is dark and has a tiny window. The eucalyptus tree is likely to suck water out from under the foundations and might render the building unstable.'

I take Deedee and Sandy to visit it as well but they agree that it's too small, and I reluctantly concede that my friends are right. I realise that Peter would have to squeeze his study into a space behind the garage, so for him it would not be a good move.

In the ensuing months I continue the search, looking at so many houses that in the end I no longer remember what I'm looking for or why, so I stop. It has become too unsettling for us all. Then that very Saturday, Deedee phones me at the bookshop.

'I've just driven past a house with an 'On Show' sign outside. It's just up the road from us and it looks wonderful from the road. Do you want to come and see it? Shall I meet you there after you close up?'

I leave the bookshop early and in haste to see the house. It's one that has always fascinated me when I've driven past it. The high white garden wall has an explosion of deep pink bougainvillea hanging over it – two huge bushes that trail down to the pavement. From the road I can see glimpses of the entrance to the house. A jacaranda tree stands sentinel by the drive, with a Namib coral tree alongside it that has bright red flowers in the winter, bunched together like a handful of fingers.

When I enter, I have the same immediate rush of excitement I had when I first saw our house on the mountain, and again I call Peter to come and see what will be our next home.

We help Alexia to buy a house of her own. Then we move away from the mountainside, from the sound of guinea fowl calling after the rain and the baboons that came to raid our fruit trees. We move into a smart, smaller house on a street that is noisy with traffic. We still have a view, but of distant hills.

This house gives me freedom. Isabel has her own bedroom with en-suite shower. Peter and I have a large bedroom and bathroom, and two small studies, side by side. Perivi has his own flat at the back and can walk or catch a taxi to the university or to see his friends. Isabel can walk to school. Both can walk to the shops to buy drinks and videos; anyone can get bread, milk or newspapers.

To fit into the new house, we have to downsize drastically. We sort out the detritus of many years of living in ample space, things never thrown away, old documents that don't need to be kept, cloths and more clothes, toys, old bicycles, old computers that work but are no longer used because they are so slow, old records from my business. I file, I box, I throw away, give away, parcel things out to different members of the family. Uazuvara is visiting once more, staying with some other friends. He comes to help and tells me that he is worried by my frenzied activity.

'It's as though you are tidying up your life before getting ready to depart from it,' he says.

The day for the move arrives – a dry, windy morning in late July 2002. Peter takes the day off work and we take carloads of small items we will need immediately, to the new house. In the afternoon, he is called to an urgent meeting but Luther is staying with us, and he helps, as he has done in the past, when I moved into the bookshop and a new office. The removal men deal with everything we don't need for the next 24 hours, because we have decided to spend the night in a guest house nearby. They don't bat an eyelid when they see the steep slope from our old house to the road, up which they must carry everything – beds, chairs, kitchen goods, clothes, books, books and more books.

The next day, as we sit on our new *stoep* after lunch and a long session of unpacking boxes, I see the smoke of a veld fire rising in the direction of the hills near the old house. I'm not alarmed, for the veld fires there always run down the back of the houses on the other side of the street, but I have an appointment at the house with an estate agent and a prospective buyer so I set off in the car.

When I turn into our old street, the smoke is thicker than I've ever seen before. I drive fast up the hill and park opposite our house, suddenly afraid of the possibility of an exploding petrol tank. I run down and through the house to the balcony. The fire is on our side of the road. It looks as if it's heading straight towards the house.

I run into the garden to turn on the sprinklers for the thatched lapa we had built last year, but the top comes off in my hand. All I can think of is that the thatch will catch fire, the whole house will burn down and, since we never got round to informing the insurance company that we had put up a thatched roof, they will not meet any claim.

I search for the garden hose to try to wet the thatch from the garden tap but it's been moved to the new house. There is water available in the swimming pool. I search for a container with which to scoop the water out. A child's plastic toy box lies in a corner of the garden shed; that's all.

I run into the house, find an abandoned telephone directory and use my cell phone to call the plumber who installed the sprinkler; he promises to come immediately. I phone Peter, and am lucky to find him still at home. I tell him to come straight over with a hose and buckets. He rushes over with Perivi and they join me in scooping up water from the pool, trying to throw it onto the thatch and the trees in the line of the fire that is now coming down the valley towards us.

The plumber arrives and manages to fix the tap and turn it on but he tells us that these sprinklers are not strong enough to stop the flames, only to dampen the thatch. The estate agent arrives with the client and I take them straight into the house. They seem unperturbed by the threat of the fire, even asking to come out onto the balcony to take a look at the view that is obscured by smoke. I leave them and go down to the garden to see how the fire is advancing. A shout comes from the estate agent:

'Water is pouring through the sitting room ceiling!'

I run back up the steps and into the house. A pipe has burst but there's nothing we can do to stop the water and nothing in the house to try to mop it up with; it just soaks into the carpet. I phone the plumber again and tell him to come back. It seems as if the house is convulsing at our departure.

The estate agent and client leave and I go back to the garden again. I look at Peter throwing water over the thatch. He checks up the valley and a sudden gust of wind sweeps the flames into the trees at the bottom of our neighbour's garden. They crackle as they head towards us.

'Run,' he shouts. 'Drop everything, just get out of here!'

Peter and Perivi run up the drive but I'm at the other side of the garden and have to run back up the steps. My legs feel heavy. At the moment I need speed, I feel as if I can hardly move, like in a bad dream. I stagger to the top. We can't see where the fire is because of the intensity of the smoke. Peter jumps into his car and drives up the hill, to get behind the fire. Perivi and I drive away down the hill and out of sight. I stop at the end of the road. I'm shaking and crying. I'm lamenting the loss of the house and the damage that could be done to our neighbours' houses as the fire jumps from our house to theirs. Perivi is shocked at my reaction. He puts his hand round my shoulder:

'It might not be as bad as you think.'

After half an hour, we return slowly back up the road, pausing where it crosses the riverbed. Blackened and smoking grass shows us that the fire has passed by; the houses are still standing. We drive back cautiously. Our old house is untouched. As we descend to the pool area, we see that, instead of jumping into our property, the fire did an abrupt turn along the course of the riverbed, which took it down below the lowest level of the garden. The sparsity of the trees there meant it did not have time to take hold and cross to the thatch. We were lucky.

Namibia was a German colony from 1884 until 1915 and this colonial past is evident in the centre of Windhoek. A sandstone neo-gothic Lutheran church with curved archways over its windows, and a spire, sits on top of the hill, looking like it came straight out of Germany. There are houses with thick walls and overhanging roofs, built during the German period, and well suited to the Namibian climate; a row of old shops with steep sloping roofs designed to allow snow to slide off, are not. An old fort right by the church, with whitewashed walls and palm trees in its central courtyard, is now a museum. A plaque on the wall at the front entrance to the fort says it was built to keep warring African communities apart. To Namibians, though, it is a symbol of German colonial power.

Behind the church, the 'Tintenpalast', which housed the German administration, has been redesigned inside to become Namibia's National Assembly, where Mosé is Speaker. A monument of a German soldier on horseback stands between the Tintenpalast and the fort. It commemorates the 1,750 Germans killed in the uprising by the Herero and Nama communities in 1904-08. There is still no monument to the estimated 60,000 Hereros and the 10,000 Namas who were slaughtered in the German response, nor to the survivors of that massacre, some of whom were confined in a concentration camp by the fort and used as forced labour to build the church and the Tintenpalast.

However, a new monument, called Heroes' Acre, has recently been built to commemorate the Namibians who fell in the struggle for independence, and I go with Peter to the inauguration on 26 August, the 36th anniversary of the launching of SWAPO's armed struggle in 1966. The monument lies on the outskirts of Windhoek, in the hills on the road south to Rehoboth. An obelisk standing 30 metres high dominates the site, as well as an 8-metre bronze statue of an unknown soldier – a bearded freedom fighter in battle fatigues holding a flaming torch high above his head. He bears a marked resemblance to the President. Behind the statue is a curved bronze relief mural telling the story of the Namibians' struggle from the time of colonial occupation: men and women fighting at first with traditional weapons, bows and arrows, and later with guns: a modern, military force. Their strong faces look familiar but are not depictions of actual people.

'I know people have criticised the statue because it looks like President Nujoma,' I say to Peter, 'and the whole style of the place is heavy. But standing here, I feel humbled by what these men and women achieved, and powerfully protected by this father of the nation.'

A slope of terraces that will become the sites for future graves rises up to the base of the obelisk. The first terrace has already been filled with memorial stones acknowledging heroes from different communities who opposed colonial rule, from the early part of the twentieth century to the start of the modern nationalist movement. Climbing the steps past these memorials, we reach the obelisk and turn to see the view. The whole of Windhoek stretches in front of us, a small town surrounded by rolling hills, brown and grey in the dryness of winter. A few patches of green from groups of trees in public and private gardens show here and there. The houses look tiny from this distance, the light glinting off their windows and corrugated iron roofs.

At the inaugural ceremony, politicians of all parties, churchmen and women, diplomats and business people gather together to name and honour these past heroes. President Nujoma gives a speech, describing the history of colonial rule and the liberation struggle, stressing that 'Heroes Acre must serve as an inspiration to our citizens, both young and old alike, that through determined and united action we can achieve our national goals…we must draw strength, inspiration and courage from this monument and all it represents.'

The Prime Minister, Hage Geingob, is the Chairman of the National Committee on Heroes' Acre, and has written a foreword to the booklet we receive on the day. In it he writes that the site commemorates 'heroes of the past, those men and women who left their mark on our Namibian heritage and who contributed to our national identity'. 'It is,' he has written, 'a dedication to all Namibians who sacrificed for others irrespective of the nature of their heroic deed.'

The first seven heroes honoured are the leaders of different communities across the country who resisted German and South African rule. Next is Chief Hosea Kutako who fought against the Germans and led the petitions to the United Nations in the late 1940s; he is considered to be the father of modern Namibian nationalism. Kakurukaze Mungunda, a woman shot and killed in the 1959 resistance to the forced removals from Windhoek's Old Location, is also honoured.

Bodily remains have been brought for reburial from the mass grave of over 600 people (mostly women and children) who were killed in the

South African attack on the Namibian settlement at Kassinga, Angola, in 1978.

Beforehand, there had been great concern about the day, about who would be remembered and who might be omitted, but it has been well thought out and well implemented. The response of people at the ceremony is positive.

The next day, we drive with Isabel, but not Perivi, to the coast for the weekend. Isabel and I are at the house when Peter comes back from the office and collects us. We get into the car and I drive off.

'I have some news to tell you,' Peter says.

'Mmm,' I respond, not paying attention. I turn on the car radio.

'In a surprise move,' says the announcer, 'President Sam Nujoma has removed Prime Minister Hage Geingob, with immediate effect. No reason has been given. At the same time, the President announced a Cabinet reshuffle.'

'That's what I wanted to tell you,' says Peter. 'I just had a call telling me about it.'

No one knows why the Prime Minister has been dismissed. We hear underlying rumours of a power struggle as to who will succeed President Nujoma. Yet the Prime Minister has served in his post since Independence. Almost everyone thinks he has done a good job and been a force for unity. We are deeply shocked by what seems an incomprehensible decision.

Two weeks later, the President lambasts British Prime Minister Tony Blair at a World Summit on Sustainable Development, over Britain's stand on Zimbabwe. Returning home, he emphasises Africa's ability to develop on its own and suggests that Namibia does not need Western aid.

Two years ago, the President had co-chaired the UN Millennium Conference that established the Millennium Development Goals, along with the then Finnish President, Tarja Halonen. Namibia's first Foreign Minister, Theo-Ben Gurirab, was the elected President of the UN General Assembly that year (1999-2000).

The Millenium Conference set targets to eliminate poverty, provide education for all, and improve health care and access to safe and affordable drinking water, by the year 2015. Namibians were so proud of the President's role. Now people are shocked by his recent actions.

We talk about it at Friday breakfast at the Brasilian. I look at Sandy, Deedee and Isobel, who were in Namibia during the days of South African rule.

'You know,' I say. 'You've lived here through bad and good times. But I've been thinking about how lucky I've been all the time I've lived in Namibia.'

I pause, and take a drink of my cappuccino.

'How d'you mean?' asks Deedee.

'I've been proud of what's happening here. I've been positive about the Government. I know you can say that this or that is not being done. I know we can argue about how to create more jobs or deal better with AIDS or provide better health and education for the people.'

I pause again. 'But I've been part of something positive, in which I could believe. These latest developments make me wonder what's going on.'

Two weeks later, I celebrate my 50th birthday in our new house. It seems like no time since I was 40, although we've been so busy in the intervening years.

'How do you feel?' my friends ask me. I'm the oldest of our breakfast group.

'It's fine. It's rather fun,' I reply. Lines are beginning to draw my mouth downwards, but I only really notice them in photos. There are wrinkles at the side of my eyes that I like; I think of them as laughter lines. My hair is greying but I streak it blonde and brown to give it more colour. There's a patch at the front, on the line of my parting that's completely white but I leave that as it is.

Uanaingi arrives in the morning of my birthday with one of our nieces, Eerike. They sort out crockery and cutlery, and make green salad, potato salad and grated carrot salad with pineapple pieces in it. They put the salads in large glass bowls, cover them in cling film and squeeze them into the fridge. Peter goes out to buy drinks and brotchen. A friend who heads the catering department at the university prepares chicken pieces, boerewors and lamb chops to braai (barbeque) later, and oryx stew in a huge pot she brings from the university that cooks slowly through the afternoon. She is the sister of Perivi's Namibian godfather, who died a few years ago.

We bring out plastic white garden tables and chairs and printed African cloths to cover them with. We arrange them round the walled courtyard at the side of the house that leads off our open-plan sitting and dining room. A separate room, with a bar, opens onto the back of the courtyard; a braai has been built into the wall at one side.

Twenty or so close family and friends gather at six in the evening, including the Friday breakfast group, Peter's sisters, his oldest son Kavesorere, with his wife and two young girls, and Uanaingi, with her daughter Diana and a new addition to her family, another daughter Utaa, now three. Two drivers from the university braai the meat. Alexia and Uanaingi put out the food. Perivi and his friends run the bar. It's the first of September, the beginning of the brief Namibian spring. The evening air is mild, the direct sun has gone and the heat that builds up in the courtyard during the day has eased.

People sit at tables with those they know, speaking English or Herero or a mixture of the two. The sounds of Hugh Masakela's music come from the CD player in the sitting room, and Clarence Carter, the African American singer. A well-known local musician and old friend, Jackson, brings his guitar and sings us songs from the old days – liberation songs that I remember from London, when we were all young. One, 'Tunana', is a praise song to the leaders of SWAPO, including Peter, calling on them to lead the people to freedom: *Tunana, tunana, k'ongutukiro.*

A Namibian friend sings along with the words and then her voice breaks and she stops. She is a former detainee, one of hundreds detained in exile in the late 1980s by SWAPO on suspicion of being South African spies. A bright young woman in her twenties then, brought down by fear, political manoeuvering and unsubstantiated accusations. No specific charges were brought against her; no evidence was offered. She was interrogated and detained but later released to take part in the independence process. No one I know has ever believed she was guilty of anything. Now she has an important public position, which may be compensation, but there's been no public acknowledgement of the wrong done to her and the shadow of that experience hangs over her.

There are other shadows as well. Tricia is about to leave Namibia, heading back to Scotland to look after her mother, although her husband Richard will remain behind. She has always felt guilty at being so far away from her mother, but she's also searching for something for herself:

better pay and professional recognition than she has had in Namibia. Now that her youngest child has finished university, she is taking the plunge and heading off on her own for a while.

Sandra is also with us. Her husband Mosé is travelling and cannot be here. It's a treat to have her with us as I don't see her often; she is always busy, bringing visitors to Namibia, promoting the country and trying to encourage investment. She has brought a friend whose husband passed away suddenly three months ago. I am conscious of other absent friends as well, and aware of how near death can be.

Normally, Peter speaks at family or social events, but tonight I decide I want to say something. I stand up, move to the centre of the courtyard, with my glass in hand, and welcome everyone. Peter comes up to stand by me.

'It's wonderful to see you all. Thank you for coming,' I say. 'I can't tell you how important it is to me to have you here. I may be far from the home I grew up in, but Namibia is my home now. You are my family. You are the ones who support me.'

I raise my glass to toast us all. 'Life is fragile,' I say. 'Let's remember each other and enjoy our time together.'

PART 2

The pit of death

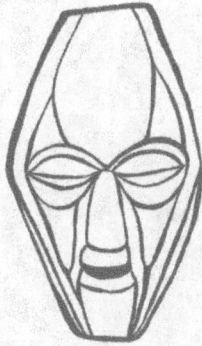

Death has stalked us this year. It began in Germany, when Luther's wife Brigitte finally lost a nine-year fight with cancer.

Brigitte and I were very close – a connection of the spirit but also of our situations – two northern European women married to wonderful but stubborn Namibian men. We loved them and occasionally complained to each other about them, without being disloyal. We understood each other's confusions or frustrations at cultural differences, even though we didn't often speak about them.

For four years, when Perivi was small and we lived in England still, we would go for holidays to their home in Bochum, northern Germany, or they would come to us. Brigitte had a son from a previous marriage, Tobias, who was a couple of years older than Perivi, and we would pair off – the two men, the two women, the two boys – and come together again later. Hot cherries over vanilla ice-cream were a favourite. Walking in the park, where the boys could play in and out of an old train engine or go on the slide – Perivi loving it even though it was very high and he was tiny. Cooking in the evenings. Dancing at home to Hugh Masakela and Barry White – Brigitte loved to dance. Talking – in English, occasional German, and Herero for the two men – and laughing. Peter laughs more with Luther than with anyone else.

Luther and Brigitte met when he went to visit a friend in Bochum, where she was living. She was teaching primary school. He was working in Nurnberg, in the south of the country, where he had moved after studying in the German Democratic Republic (GDR). For a couple of years, they commuted to see each other at the weekends. She thought of moving to join him but it was difficult for teachers to transfer from one German state to another, so eventually Luther gave up his job and moved to Bochum to be with her.

She went to Namibia before Independence, a few years before I did, deciding that she needed to see Luther's country and meet his family, even though he couldn't go with her because of his involvement with SWAPO.

'On the plane there,' she told me after her return, 'the man next to me asked where I would be staying. I said with my brother-in-law. He asked me where that was. So I said "Katutura". He looked as if he couldn't believe it, because he knew it must mean that my husband is black and because whites in Namibia never go to Katutura– they are too afraid.'

It was the mid-1980s, a time when there was a build-up of student protests and suppression of them by the South African authorities, but Brigitte's stay was peaceful. Luther's brother Obed met her at the airport and took her to his home.

'The house was better than many of the houses in Katutura,' she said, 'and although it's small, I had my own room, and neighbours and family members came to see me. I met Peter's sister and her daughters. Obed showed me round. We went to Etosha, and he took me to Ovitoto, to Okasuvandjiuo, to meet their mother, Inaa; their sisters; and Kutji, their elder brother. We spoke in German. Everyone was friendly. I loved it. I didn't really want to come back home.'

She showed us her photos – relatives that Peter and Luther have not seen for more than 20 years, new babies, the animals in Etosha, Brigitte milking a cow, and in a Herero dress with Luther's mother.

'Which road did you take to go to Ovitoto?' Peter wanted to know. He and Luther didn't recognise it from the photo. 'Where is it in relation to the river?'

'You cross the river and go past the school and then you have to drive over bare rock because the road disappears,' she replied, but the road was new and they could not quite locate it, trying to compare her photos with their memories of the place they had left over 20 years before.

We went to Brigitte and Luther's wedding the following year, a civil ceremony in Bochum with Brigitte wearing a full-skirted turquoise blue dress – a big change from her usual jeans and polo shirts. Her parents and grandfather were there, with us and five other Namibians. We went on for a meal at a restaurant nearby, followed by a more informal get-together with friends in their flat in the evening. She showed me the Herero dress she had been given by Luther's mother. We both tried it on and took photos of each other in it, looking very alike – white faces and big glasses, short hair hidden by the *otjikaeva* headdress.

Brigitte was an only child and Tobias her parents' only grandchild. She felt a great sense of responsibility to stay close to them. She had been living, literally, on top of her parents, in the same apartment block, two stories above, and Luther moved in with her there. It wasn't easy for him because Brigitte's mother was so involved in Brigitte's life. She was house-proud in a traditional German way, believing that there was only one way of doing things. Luther clashed with her often.

After we moved to the USA and then to Namibia, Brigitte and I saw each other rarely, only when they came from Bochum to visit us. In 1993, she was diagnosed with breast cancer. At the time, Peter was intensely busy in the early days of establishing the university. I was intensely busy in the early days of my publishing, and juggling that with the demands of young children. We didn't get over to Germany to see them and I often felt that I didn't talk to her enough or give her enough support at the time.

Brigitte had endless treatments, various operations, different bouts of chemotherapy, and continued life as normally as possible.

'I think about it every day,' she told me. It was always with her, the possibility that the cancer might still be there, somewhere, waiting to come back and strike again, which is what it did, one year after her six-year check-up when she had been declared cancer-free.

This time it started with an ache in her left arm, a little difficulty in lifting it, during one of her visits to Namibia (it would be her last). I don't know the exact cause; don't know whether it was the fluid building up because of drainage problems after the lymph glands under her arm on that side had been excised. But the fluid came later, bloating her arm, and making it almost impossible for her to lift it.

She went through another course of chemotherapy, and responded well. We grew hopeful again, believing that the cancer could be kept at bay. Luther kept faith. Brigitte stayed positive, reduced her teaching hours and took up painting, and singing in a local choir. Was there anyone to whom she confided her deepest fears, or had she already entered that zone where the sick protect the healthy from what they know is happening?

After another year, Brigitte grew weaker. She stopped work completely to concentrate on her health. She willed Tobias to do well in his final school exams and willed herself to keep going as long as possible to support him. She held on, and held on, and held on, until her son had finished school and she could hold on no longer.

Towards the end, as Brigitte's health really started to fail, I sent her emails to which she had no strength to reply. I spoke to Luther on the phone and he made it clear that she was terribly ill. I phoned one day from the bookshop and had to roll the chair back and hide behind one of the stacks as my tears flowed while I talked. I needed to get out of sight so that I could let my feelings out, away from my usual place in full view of people as they came through the door.

Just before the end of December, I flew to Germany to see them, knowing that I would be saying goodbye to her.

I entered the flat, hung up my coat, took off my outside shoes, and slipped into a pair of the many house shoes lined up by the door. Then I went in to greet Brigitte. She had been sitting in a big armchair with her legs up but she was on her feet now, walking slowly across the room to meet me.

'Sisi, I'm sorry,' I said and hugged her gently. 'How are you doing?'

Brigitte smiled: 'I am so happy you're here, and you came – all this way – just to see me.'

We stayed most of the time in their flat or went downstairs to her parents for lunch – Brigitte's mother was now cooking for them every day. Luther and I did the shopping and went for a few walks. The cold winter air was a welcome contrast to the centrally heated apartment that I found difficult after the open-air living of Namibia.

Although Brigitte needed to rest a lot, we talked, listened to music together (this time Strauss, not Masakela) and watched a little television. We caught two programmes about Namibia. One was about Sandy's production of 'Lysistrata' and another on the work of the Cheetah Conservation Fund, set up by an American woman, Laurie Marker, and with which I am involved. I was reminded once again how courageous these women are.

Each morning, Brigitte's mother, now in her early eighties, came up the two flights of stairs, to wash and dress Brigitte. A nurse who lived in the flat immediately below came most days as well, to gently massage Brigitte's swollen arm and try to keep the fluids from building up even more.

On New Year's Eve we planned a special meal.

'Rabbit in red wine sauce,' said Brigitte. 'You and Luther can cook and I'll tell you what to do.'

I chopped while Luther did most of the cooking. Then I laid the table, around which we had sat so many times with Peter as well, eating late breakfasts and early dinners, Perivi and Tobias in the room next door. Tobi's first English words were put to regular practice to stop the younger Perivi playing too boisterously with his toys:

'Pereevi, don't do it!'

At the window, later, we watched fireworks set off in neighbouring gardens and street corners to celebrate and welcome in 2002.

I never told Brigitte how much I loved her but she knew. I never talked about whether or not this was the end but we both knew that her end was near. She didn't give up. With the courage of so many who are seriously ill, she faced each day with dignity and without complaint. She smiled, she laughed and she participated as much as she could.

When I left, it was Luther who needed comforting. He was still trying desperately to believe that Brigitte would survive. But a month later she was in hospital again and two weeks after that she died. As soon as I heard his voice on the phone, I knew. I was flooded with a terrible mixture of grief and relief. The words of Martin Luther King in his 'I Have a Dream' speech came to me: 'Free at last, free at last, thank God Almighty, she is free at last.' You do not want people you love to suffer, to collapse slowly and painfully, to be eaten up by disease as well as by the medication taken to try to defeat it. She had already suffered long and hard enough.

In Windhoek, we phoned friends and relatives, put notices on the radio and in the newspaper. Her funeral was a quiet family affair in Bochum and we held a memorial service at the university on the same day. Getting it organised gave me something useful to do. Friends and family came; some of them knew Brigitte well, others were there largely to support us. It gave us the opportunity to speak of her, of our love for her, and to pay tribute to her. Isobel was there, along with Deedee and Sandy, Uazuvara (Bente was away), Sandra and many others.

We played music from a CD recorded by the choir that Brigitte had belonged to. Somewhere in that swell of sound, was her voice. I read a passage from the Society of Friends Guide:

> Death is not an end, but a beginning. It is but an incident in the 'life of the ages', which is God's gift to us *now*. It is the escape of the spirit from its old limitations and its freeing for a larger and more glorious career. We stand around the grave, and as we take our last, lingering look, too often our thoughts are *there*; and we return to the desolate home feeling that all that made life lovely has been left behind on the bleak hillside... Yet the spirit now is *free*, and the unseen angel at

our side points upwards from the grave and whispers, 'She is not here, but is risen'. The dear one returns with us to our home, ready and able, as never before, to comfort, encourage, and beckon us onward.

'I like that,' Isobel said. 'It's beautiful.'

Six months later, in August 2002, sitting at the back of the bookshop one Saturday morning, chatting to Peter on the phone, I opened my emails and glanced across them. One announced the assassination of Chief Victor Nwankwo, a Nigerian publisher and friend. As I took in the news, I could no longer breathe. Peter heard me gasp and called out down the phone. I couldn't speak. I shoved the phone at Doris so that she could communicate with Peter, but he had already left the café where he was enjoying a glass of champagne and a brotchen with Uazuvara, and was running through the streets towards the bookshop. He arrived a few minutes later as I was collecting myself.

Victor was a close colleague. I had worked with him on the Board of the African Publishers' Network (APNET) and saw him regularly at book fairs across the continent. He was a gentle, meticulous, humorous man dedicated to developing publishing in Africa. Brother of a flamboyant public political figure, he ran the family publishing business in Enugu, eastern Nigeria. He had fought as a young man on the Biafran side of the civil war, and sometimes spoke of the famine and misery at the end of the war, when a million Igbos died.

I emailed publishing colleagues, to share the information and to try to find out more. It transpired that Victor had been gunned down outside his house one night as he returned home. Fellow publishers believe he was killed because he was about to publish a book exposing corruption in his state.

I last saw Victor at the Zimbabwe International Book Fair one month before he was killed, and said goodbye to him the evening before I was due to fly home, watching him walk off to his room, hands in the pockets of the baggy trousers of his cotton Nigerian suit, chuckling at what we had been talking about. We had spent the evening together, five or six or us, discussing publishing and Zimbabwe, and laughing at the idea of a mock memorial for the mosquito in West Africa, which had kept white settlers out of the area and so prevented the sort of land and racial problems that Zimbabwe was experiencing.

I heard about Victor's death a few days before my 50th birthday. Now, six weeks later, I prepare to go to his funeral, delayed by the attempts to get a proper investigation into his death. This will be my first ever visit to Nigeria. I had told Victor some years ago that I would love to see his country.

'It's not a good time to visit Nigeria,' he had said, 'the country still suffering under the Abacha military regime. 'Come when we have a democratic government. Then you can also come home.'

APNET's last General Assembly had been held in the Nigerian capital, Abuja, earlier in the year, in recognition of the fact that Nigeria had now achieved a democratic government, but I could not go because it clashed with Patji's wedding. I never dreamt that when I went got to Nigeria it would be for Victor's funeral.

I have been asked by APNET to represent southern Africa at the funeral and I fly to Johannesburg and meet the APNET Executive Secretary and the Acting Director of the Zimbabwe International Book Fair there. We fly together to Lagos. My mind is full of the comments people make about Nigeria, about being asked for 'extra pages' (dollar notes) in your passport, about overcrowded towns and cities, and creative crime, cut across with memories of working with Victor and how much I learned from him about publishing and institutional development.

I had packed four cotton African dresses, some light shawls and a spare pair of sandals, and carried the bag with me on the plane because I didn't want to risk losing my suitcase. But when we arrive, our passage through passport control and customs is without incident, the airport modern and efficient. We transfer to a domestic terminal to fly to Enugu in the east of Nigeria. For four months in 1967, Enugu was the capital of the breakaway state of Biafra. Then, when Nigerian federal forces retook it, the town of Umuahia became the Biafran capital until just before the end of the civil war two years later. Peter studied in Umuahia from 1964 to 1966 on a scholarship given by the Nigerian government through SWAPO, not long after he had left Namibia and gone into exile. He was at the Government Training College, where the curriculum included Latin and an officer training corps under the leadership of Chief Ojukwu, who went on to lead the Biafran forces.

Enugu looks as if it was once an attractive city, but the buildings are in need of repair. They look run down and dirty from the red laterite soil that heavy rains have splashed onto them over the years. The side roads are full of potholes. Trees and bushes push through urban spaces, the richness of the environment completely different from our sparse Namibian landscapes. In our hotel, the bedrooms have en-suite bathrooms. Full-size plastic dustbins standing in the bath are filled

84

with water for us each day; it's tepid so it doesn't matter that there is no running hot and cold water.

Other APNET and African publishing colleagues are at the same hotel and we go together to visit Victor's family at their home to offer our condolences. We sit with Victor's wife Oby, a lawyer who is very involved in the community and in issues of women's rights. She tells us more about what happened.

'I was at home and I heard gunfire, very near our house. I tried to phone Victor to tell him to be careful because it was about the time he usually came home, but there was no answer from his cell phone. The guard decided to go out of the compound. He saw a police car driving down the street. Victor was in his car just outside the house. He had been shot point blank. We took him to the hospital and I stayed with him there through the night. The police came and harassed me, telling me that I must go home. I refused. I didn't know what they might do to Victor. But we couldn't save him.'

Victor was not a politician but he was critical of the state government, and his family view his killing as political. It has been followed by other killings in the eastern states – two lawyers, and a university professor.

Victor and Oby's children are at school and college in the USA, living with family members. They have travelled over for the funeral and come in to greet us. I go to their 20-year-old son.

'I want you to know how much we respected your father. He was a wonderful man. He talked about you all a lot. I have a son a little younger than you. Your father met him once, and he gave my son a nickname – Mr Cool.'

'I didn't really know my father,' he replied. He had been away so long.

We visit Fourth Dimension, the publishing house where Victor had pioneered the digital development and storing of books sent as files to the UK for printing and export sales. In contrast to this high-tech side of the business, the road to his office is in a terrible mess, full of potholes, muddy and slippery after the rain.

A service at the Anglican Church in Enugu starts the two-day funeral programme and afterwards the convoy of hearse, cars and buses passes through the town, stopping at the Fourth Dimension offices for people to say farewell to Victor. The hearse is decorated with a banner reading 'Transition to Glory'. The convoy of those who are going on to the burial continues to Victor's home village, Ajalli, a few hours' drive to the east. We pass through forest and green cultivated fields but I don't recognise the crops. We pause at the entrance to the village for a gun salute and then proceed to the family compound.

The visitors are given accommodation at different homes in the village. Two other APNET colleagues and I are driven to a house in the forest. It's already getting dark and on the way, we bump over a large snake on the road. We are each given a room; we freshen up and then return to the family compound. Bottled water, cool drinks and plates of stew and vegetables are provided for us.

Over 800 people come for the wake-keeping that goes on through much of the night, with drumming, dance and masquerade. As visitors, we are invited to join in, but I don't want to. I don't want to dance at Victor's funeral.

'We must give him a good send off,' I'm told. 'This is the way we show how much we cared.'

There are over 1000 at the church service and burial the next day, including family members, friends, church leaders, local community elders, African and international publishers, Nigerian chiefs, the Governor of the neighbouring state, and the former leader of Biafra, Chief Ojukwu. Then Victor is buried in the compound of the family home.

His brother issues a press statement on the day of the burial, laying the blame for the killing squarely on the authorities of the local state. At the final church service in Ajalli, the priest says 'Do not weep for Victor. Weep for yourselves and for your children. Weep for Nigeria.'

On my return to Windhoek, I apply myself to marketing workshops with upper primary school teachers in the densely populated north of Namibia. The workshops focus on the use of English-language fiction and non-fiction readers in schools, and are held at educational circuit offices. There are 16 such circuits to cover and I hold two or three during a week's visit. The workshop outline I use was prepared by the publishers we represent and adapted by me to the local situation and context, but I am on my own in the preparation and delivery.

I write to the circuit inspector to arrange the workshops, write to the schools, prepare the workshop, make necessary changes, choose the books we will work on and select passages from them, book the hotel, and buy the refreshments for participants. I drive north for two and a half hours and pick up one of our nephews, Munionganda, at the town of Otjiwarongo. He helps me with the driving and takes me the rest of the way (another four hours), to Ondangwa.

'How are your parents?' I ask him (his mother is one of Luther's sisters).

'Fine.'

'And how are things on the farm?'

'Good.'

'Did you get enough rain there this year?'

'Not bad.'

'I hear you're getting married.'

'Yes.'

When will the wedding be?'

'December.'

He doesn't talk much but he's helpful and it's good to have someone with me.

This part of Namibia is a flat flood plain, with sandy soil, woodlands in some areas and makalani palm trees in others. A water system of drainage channels runs south from Angola, creating *oshanas* – pools where the water gathers – that are used by people and animals until they dry out; then water becomes a problem. This Cuvelai drainage network leads into the Etosha Pan, heart of the Etosha game reserve. I've visited this area before, but not very often. Now, we explore parts I've never been to, finding our way down sandy lanes and through *mahangu* (millet) fields. Driving back at the end of the day, the sun shines low through the grass, giving it a golden glow. It's a beautiful but fragile landscape.

This is the most densely populated part of Namibia, quite unlike the centre and south of the country. Circular fenced traditional homesteads with thatched huts and five-foot-high woven grain baskets stand in the middle of the *mahangu* fields. Modern, brick-built houses appear between them. Tin roofed roadside bars sport names like 'Club Put More Fire'; they first appeared to serve the South African army who were in this area in the 1970s and 1980s, fighting against SWAPO.

The circuit offices are new and purpose-built since Independence for meetings of teachers and inspectors, and for training seminars. They are single-storey buildings with corrugated iron roofs, and contain the inspector's office and usually two large rooms, with 20 or 30 chairs in them. There is air conditioning in only one of the circuit offices I visit.

'We didn't have any money for it in the budget,' the circuit inspector tells me. 'But I suggested it to the teachers. I pointed out that it was in their interest to have one, and they each contribute a few dollars at month-end when they are paid, to cover the cost.'

At the beginning of each workshop, the teachers gather slowly and take a cool drink from the supply I provide. They have come on from their lessons, at the end of their normal school day, catching lifts with others. It is early afternoon, the worst time for concentration, but most of them are keen. They teach pupils who must learn to speak English even though they hardly hear it, except perhaps on television for those in the towns and peri-urban areas where there's electricity.

When I first visited schools in this area eight years ago, I couldn't believe that pupils walk up to 15 kilometres to school, where there is sometimes no water to revive them, bringing little or no food or drink, and then have to focus on the work before them. I couldn't communicate with many of the teachers because they didn't speak English. They could hardly use the textbooks that had been approved by the Ministry that were in English.

Too many pupils still walk long distances to and from school. We pass them on their dusty walks home after school has finished, while we are driving to the education circuit offices. What's different now is that English has spread, and the teachers' knowledge of it is much greater. I can get around more easily but the schools still have too few learning materials.

I deliver the workshops to 20-plus teachers at a time. We look at different uses of the readers, for specific subject content and for cross-curricular activities and language work. The stories themselves are fun; the non-fiction readers well thought-out and well designed. The teachers enjoy working with them and share ideas from their own experiences, but I don't know if they can use this in their work without the books. My job is to close the workshop with a sales pitch, trying to persuade them to request the books from their principals. This is the part I dislike as I know the schoolbook budgets are too small.

At the hotel after the workshop, I go to my room, kick off my shoes, lie on the bed and drink Coke, relishing the sugar and the caffeine after a hot and tiring afternoon. I write up a short report about the workshop. My lunch is a sandwich, so I go for dinner in the hotel dining room, choosing steak and chips or meat stew with spinach and rice, a glass of red wine and a lot of water. Sometimes Munionganda joins me for the meal, but not always. I return to my room, watch the news on TV and go to bed.

At the end of a week delivering the workshops, I return to Windhoek feeling exhausted but I have no time to rest, because I have to turn my attention to the financial record keeping. I'm convinced that the workshops will increase sales and keep my business going, and I push myself to continue them, but they are a punishing schedule to add to my duties at the bookshop.

On one trip to the north, I wake in the night after delivering a workshop that day, shivering, although it's not cold. I have a bad headache and my stomach is cramping painfully. I open the window to try to get some air, checking to make sure there are no holes in the mosquito netting across it. The only noise outside is the whirr of air conditioners in other rooms nearby (mine did not work and in any case I don't like sleeping with them on). I swallow two paracetamol, drink a bottle of water, and try to get back to sleep. In the morning, I feel tired and slow and I still have stomach ache. I eat some porridge and drink black tea, wondering if it's something I have eaten that's upset me.

Munionganda and I drive to a circuit office 40 kilometres from the hotel and I deliver another workshop to a small group of teachers – only nine this time, since the circuit inspector has not been active bringing in teachers from the schools in his district. He has double-booked the larger classroom so we make do with a small room that is half full of boxes of paper and other school supplies. I don't have the energy to make much effort to enthuse the teachers; I just want the workshop to be over. When it is, we head home. I drop Munionganda at Otjiwarongo to go back to the farm where he looks after his parents' cattle and I overnight there in a small hotel. I get up before six next morning to drive to Windhoek in time for a meeting but when I arrive, I feel so tired that I rearrange the meeting and go home to bed.

When I have a heavy cold and feel too sick to work, I take two days off and go to bed. I hide from the world, drink a lot of tea, and read. It usually works. So I take two days off now and think I'm taking care of myself. On the second night an acute pain across my chest wakes me up; it's unlike anything I've ever experienced. It's too high to be anything to do with my stomach and too sharp to be the dull ache of bronchitis, with which I'm familiar. I turn in one direction, then the other, and onto my back to try to see if that will stop it, but it makes no difference. I try to breathe through it but it doesn't stop. I've never experienced a pain as intense as this. I look at my watch and after five minutes with no change I think 'I have to get to hospital'. Just as I'm about to wake Peter and ask him to take me, the pain disappears. I lie awake for an hour wondering what caused it and eventually drift back to sleep. The next day I tell Doris about it.

'Maybe it's anxiety,' she says, and I put it out of my mind.

A month later, I fall ill again. I wake in the night with my head throbbing, acute stomach ache, stiff and cramped in fetal position, curled on my right side. My heart bangs away against the mattress when I lie on my left. I call the bookshop to say I won't be in and ask Doris to open up for me. I stay at home for a few days and rest but I cannot shake this off. I go to the doctor who arranges various tests to try to establish what's wrong. I return to my bed and lie there, not even reading. I play classical music I haven't listened to in years. I dig out a recording of Fauré's Requiem and listen to it repeatedly, feeling desperately sad.

One morning, as I get up, I feel I'm going to collapse. I phone the doctor. The tests she has done have not revealed anything, so she suggests that I go to hospital for more extensive ones. Foul things to drink, foul instruments are used to search my body. A CT scan of the liver suggests that my pancreas looks a bit funny. I have dull pains in that area, but not acute ones. I lie in bed in the hospital, sinking into fear that this is something really serious. I fear decay. I pray that I don't have cancer and won't slowly disintegrate in pain and suffering over a period of years, as did Brigitte.

I have a room to myself so there's little noise from other patients or their visitors, but I can hear the nurses moving up and down the corridor, occasionally calling to each other. They come in on their rounds to check my blood pressure and pulse. Family and friends come with flowers, and one morning I wake to see Isobel sitting by my side. She takes my hand.

'I wanted to see how you are doing but I didn't want to wake you. I just popped in to say hello.' She chats for a while about her children and then leaves.

My blood pressure is low, my pulse is low, but nothing serious is found. I am discharged and told to come back in six months for another CT scan if the symptoms persist. A suggestion that stress might be a factor hangs between Peter and the physician. I leave the hospital with instructions about what to eat and what not to eat, and advice about getting enough rest.

The days off work have made me less, not more, inclined to go back. I start arriving later at the bookshop and leave more for Doris to deal with in the afternoons. But I have started something by talking to her about wanting to give it all up.

'We're taking stock of our situation,' she tells me. 'Clive is at retirement age, I'm doing three jobs and bills keep piling up. I also want to get away from it all.' She pauses.

'We're thinking of looking for somewhere else to live, in semi-retirement, where we could buy a house outright.' They could put the years of mortgage repayments behind them.

'We started looking at the options but you know what it's like. The cheaper places are in the small towns but what would we do there? Then there's Swakop, where the prices are not much cheaper than in Windhoek, and Clive's pension isn't large.'

They begin to look further afield. They consult South African friends about different places in the Cape, and decide that's where they will go, the cost of living (outside Cape Town) being much lower than in Windhoek. It will be a new start, although they will not be entirely alone; they have friends and Clive's brother in South Africa, and their youngest son is studying in Cape Town. They search the internet, exploring different towns, and put in an offer for a house in Ceres, a market town in a valley of fruit trees and fruit juice production, behind the mountain ranges outside Cape Town.

'I've been here 35 years, you know,' Doris says as we have a glass of wine after closing the bookshop one day. 'I was 16 when I left Frankfurt. My adult life has been here in Namibia. My children were born here. My parents died here. So much of me is tied up with this place. I shall miss Namibia. I shall miss you, my friend.'

I am horrified at the idea of her going away but I'm also jealous of her having the courage to make such a big change.

'I'll miss you too. I'll miss our long conversations. I'll miss your knowledge of my history here, right from when I first arrived. I don't know what I would have done without you then, with Peter so busy. And it's been so good working with you in the bookshop.'

But the process of making the decision to leave prompts Doris's unraveling. So much is now up in the air, so much unclear. Then comes the day when she does not come to work. I phone the house and am told she isn't feeling well. The next day it's the same, and the next. Eventually I speak to her and ask what's wrong.

'I started crying and could not stop.'

The anti-depressants she is prescribed need two weeks to take effect and even then she is excruciatingly vulnerable. Somehow in that confusion of misery and medication, Doris packs up their lives, one box per day, and tells the children they will have to learn to look after themselves. She and Clive move to a simpler life in the Cape.

Without Doris to develop the bookshop with me, and given my reduced energy levels, I decide not to renew the shop lease that expires soon. I will concentrate on the marketing, which could bring in more income from commissions than the shop, with less administration required.

'It seems terrible,' I tell Peter. 'I feel I've failed. First the publishing, now this. I loved the bookshop so much at the beginning but I just don't want to do it anymore.' I often tell him to give things up, to lessen the demands on him, but Peter never gives up on anything, a quality of commitment he learned from his Aunt Maria.

'Never turn back,' she taught him. 'When you've started a journey, you continue, you don't turn back.'

'Better that you should do something you enjoy,' he says to me now. 'You don't have to do the same thing forever.'

I agree to sell the stock to someone else who wants to start a bookshop, with a different profile but carrying some similar titles. I put other books on sale. I give away samples and slightly damaged books to school libraries.

The rhythm and ritual of our Friday breakfasts sustains me as my friends encourage me and give advice. But we are finding that the breakfast meetings are not enough. Once we start talking, we don't want to stop. We switch to having breakfast at each other's homes rather than at the Brasilian, rotating round different houses, so that it isn't a burden on any one of us. It means that we can sit for longer without feeling guilty about not appearing at our places of work, because we're not in public. We are less noisy and more relaxed than in town.

Deedee provides fruit juice and delicious muffins, croissants and jam. We sit on her balcony, with a view of the hills of Ludwigsdorf, and watch the long-tailed mouse birds in the camelthorn trees around her house.

'How are you feeling, Jane-Jane?' my namesake asks.

'Tired.' I say. 'And apart from being tired, I'm also worried about my dear son. He's not enjoying the course he's doing at UNAM and, quite honestly, I'm not sure that he's even going to his classes.'

'What doesn't he like about it?' Isobel asks.

'It's media and communications but the first-year courses are very general ones, to bring people up to the same level. He's bored and demotivated.'

'What does he want to do?'

'All he's ever wanted is to make films, since he was about eight. We thought this would be a good stepping-stone but now he's decided to leave.'

'Perhaps he's depressed,' suggests Isobel. 'We have a good friend who's a psychologist if you're interested.'

'I'm sure it will work out alright,' says Deedee. 'He just has to work out how to do what he wants to do.'

'He's creative!' Sandy exclaims. 'He needs a more creative environment.'

I think that they are all partly right.

'Find him some lovely liberal arts college,' says Deedee, 'I'm a great believer in liberal arts degrees. Then he can go on from there to film school.'

'He says he wants to go to the UK to work.' I respond. 'He has Namibian friends working in London already and he wants to stay with them. It sounds silly, but I'm worried that he will get lost in such a big city. At least in Windhoek we know what he's doing and where he might be.'

At Isobel's, we sit in the garden that dips down into a riverbed, with no real border fence. It's mid-December, the height of the hot season, and even though it's early we sit in the shade. She has laid out fruit, coffee, tea, bread and muffins, and boiled eggs.

It's the first time I have been to Isobel's house because I haven't known her as long as the others. It is a compact, artistic space designed by Hugo, the rooms full of interesting pictures, including some that Isobel has painted.

'I have to tell you, I'm really fed up,' opens Deedee.

'Why?' 'With what?' we ask.

'We've just had a visit from some more development advisers,' she continues. 'Okay, we all know there's so much we couldn't do without donor support. But some of the advisers! They come here, knowing almost nothing about Namibia, but they have the power to choose projects, to make or break them. They don't like to take advice from people on the ground. They don't look for or listen to local knowledge and experience. Everything is still determined by the ideas and priorities of the donor. There's a trend – this time it might be rural communities, or education, or HIV/AIDS – and then that changes and the projects that have been depending on that support are left high and dry.'

'And the language,' she goes on. 'The terminology. There are certain buzzwords, catch phrases that have to be used in a project description for it to get approval, and certain concepts of measuring success. They, too, change with the fashion!'

Bente joins in: 'I agree. We should start with the needs of Namibian communities and ask them where they want help. What is development after all? It has to come from the people, otherwise we only make them dependent, we don't empower them.'

I think some development experts are the new missionaries in Africa – outsiders coming to tell the locals what to believe and how to behave. But I should be careful because we too have come from outside.

We discuss the meaning of development and how it can be achieved. We discuss the role of NGOs and government, the needs of Namibian communities. We are at our best. I feel lucky to be part of such a group. Afterwards, I regret that I did not have a camera to catch us together that day. I plan to take one with me the next time. But there is no next time.

As they have done so many times before, Sandy, Deedee and Isobel go to the coast with their families for the long summer holiday. They prepare for a Christmas meal together at Langstrand, a growing residential development between Swakopmund and Walvis Bay, where Isobel and Hugo have a small bungalow in a tiered complex looking out to the open sea. There is sand all around, the sand of the beach and also the sand of the desert that comes right down to the ocean. The sea itself is silver-grey under the coastal cloud or dark greeny blue when the sun comes out, but always the colour of cold water.

Langstrand was a real Afrikaner place before Independence, and still is to some extent. As part of the Walvis Bay port area, it had been excluded from Namibia's Independence agreement. It was finally returned to Namibia along with Walvis Bay in 1994, shortly before South Africa's first free all-race elections. It was in Langstrand that Peter and I and our children were refused a table at a restaurant one year after Independence, because it was still deemed to be part of South Africa and still whites-only. That was a time when all travellers had to show their passports and get a South African stamp in them just to travel the 30 kilometres from Swakopmund to Walvis Bay.

While Hugo goes down to the coast with their two children, Isobel stays in Windhoek till the last possible moment, to finish work she's doing as a consultant on a new law that will govern the Medical Council; then she joins the family. On Christmas Day, she, Deedee, Sandy and another friend, Denise, have a midday drink together. They are relaxed and happy, sitting in deckchairs in the sunshine, sunglasses on against the bright light reflected by the sea.

A few hours later, the world turns. Out of the blue, as she prepares her part of the meal, Isobel has a heart attack and collapses. Alone in the house while others are out, she is found by Deedee who goes to check on her. They rush her to hospital and then she is flown to Cape Town, to a hospital specialising in cardiac care.

A few days later, I speak to Isobel on the phone in her hospital room. I'm surprised that her voice sounds quite strong.

'They tell me I have a failed heart,' she says. 'This is something I will have to learn to live with. I'll have to change my life, but I can do that. I just want to be able to live a bit longer, even just one year, for the children.'

Hugo flies to Cape Town with Isobel, leaving their children – Jan Barend and Kara – in Namibia in the care of friends in Windhoek. Her mother, brothers and sisters, relatives and other friends in South Africa travel to see her in hospital. Once her condition has stabilised, Hugo returns to Windhoek for the children and they go together to Cape Town to collect Isobel and bring her home. When they arrive at the hospital, she is waiting just inside the door to greet them, dressed because she wants to spare the children the distress of seeing her in a hospital bed. They sit and talk. Then she spends one last night in the hospital while the others go to a nearby hotel.

In the morning, Hugo leaves early to fetch Isobel. They sit in the doctor's consulting room, Isobel ready to be discharged. She talks about the changes to her lifestyle that she knows are necessary to try to cope with the damage to her heart and to avoid further attacks. As the doctor is reassuring her, she says she doesn't feel very well. Her heart gives up and she is gone.

They clear the doctor's rooms so it becomes a private family area. Isobel's body is laid out on the examination couch and they go and sit beside her. Hugo remembers how he was not able to say goodbye properly to his own father when he died, and he asks that they be given enough time with Isobel. Jan Barend sits with the pale, pained stillness of adolescence. Kara climbs up onto the bed and lies beside her mother, talking to her occasionally, picking up her hand, stroking her face, willing life back into her, until she can accept that the body is just that, and her mother has gone from it.

Isobel's funeral is as extraordinary as Victor's but in a different way. It starts with a service at the chapel in the cemetery in Pioneers Park, near the Old Location cemetery where people killed during the resistance to the forced removals in 1959 are buried. Surrounded by cedar trees, it has a sense of peace that struck me strongly the first time I ever went there; it left me knowing that is where I want to be buried. I almost brought my sister to see the place when she came to visit, wanting her to know where I would one day be laid to rest.

For Isobel, the small chapel is full with over 200 people – friends and some of their children, teachers from the schools where her children go, colleagues from the legal community, including the Ministry of Justice and the Office of the Attorney General.

The funeral is extraordinary because everything is organised and conducted by family and friends. Hugo is anxious about having a religious ceremony, as he and Isobel have been burned by the Calvinist heritage of their people and try to avoid it. He asks a friend who is a priest to conduct the service and plans it for the afternoon to give the priest time to drive over from Botswana, but he has car problems and cannot make it. So it falls to Deedee's husband, Michael, to lead the service. Michael is an unusual churchman, a priest with a motorbike, full of energy, direct and impatient at times, focused on the economic and social, as well as spiritual upliftment of people. He is no longer a parish priest but is in charge of a youth enterprise centre he set up that gives young Namibians vocational training to help them earn a living. Now he has to preside over Isobel's burial and try to comfort the rest of us.

There is one eulogy, written by Hugo and read by Michael. It captures the many dimensions of Isobel, speaking openly and freely about different aspects of her life. In it, Hugo speaks about her visit to her father and how that had resolved many old conflicts. He speaks about her joy at her children, and the many months she had to lie in a hospital bed before Kara was born, because she was at risk of losing the baby. ('Kara' means 'stay' in Herero, but they didn't know that then.) He speaks about how much Isobel gave to friends and family, how she didn't hesitate to confront foolishness and injustice. He tells us that she was excited about what this new year might hold for her. They had just been to Katima Mulilo in the Caprivi to experience the full solar eclipse and he saw it as 'a symbol of the brief spell of darkness which is death, followed by a reawakening to the music of birds and gentle light all around'.

'When she was in Cape Town,' Hugo continues, 'following her heart attack, she told us that she was no longer uncomfortable with the idea of death, that it was simply a door through which she will pass one day, and she remarked that at least there will be one familiar smiling face on the other side, waiting for the rest of us when we get there.' He reassures us that she died peacefully and painlessly.

It is not until I hear the eulogy that I understand what an important role Isobel played in drafting legislation in Namibia. She was responsible for drafting close to 50 new laws and amendments, some of which were unique in the Southern African legal context. Equally significant, she drafted the very first government notice for Namibia, to establish the Legal Services Commission. This in turn made it possible for our first President to be sworn in.

A black and white reproduction of a self-portrait Isobel painted a couple of years earlier has been printed on the service sheet. In it, Isobel's eyes are closed, her face an extraordinary mask.

'You know, that's exactly how Isobel looked when I went to view the body,' Deedee tells me when she sees the service sheet. What had Isobel foreseen?

To me, though, the most extraordinary thing about Isobel's funeral is the boys. I had heard that Jan Barend and his friends might be pallbearers and I was horrified at the idea of them taking on this task at such a young age. Now I see them coming with her coffin down the side-aisle at the end of the service. Her husband Hugo, her youngest brother, and Jan Barend and his friends – the sons of Deedee and Sandy – 16-year-olds made men this day.

They carry her coffin to the hearse. Hugo and Jan Barend go round the mourners and thank them all for coming. As the light begins to change in the late afternoon, we drive through town into the hills surrounding Windhoek.

At the beginning of the year, when the rains start and there are clouds in the sky, the usual brightness is shot across with shadow. Late afternoon, early evening, as the sun goes down, the angles of shadow, light and dark, lie across the land. We have had early rain this year and the hills are already turning green. Hugo has chosen a koppie – a rocky outcrop – on the family farm of their closest friends, where Isobel can lie and survey the land around her. Picture the vastness of Namibia, out beyond the capital, where there is nothing except open hills and farmland and the occasional farmhouse and buildings. We drive in 4x4s from the farmhouse to the koppie, a high point with a 360-degree view. I feel as if I can see the whole of Africa.

The grave has been carved out of the stone hilltop. About 30 of us sing favourite hymns and Michael performs the interment rites. In one direction the clouds burst and I can see the rain descending on one part of the farm, although we remain dry. Behind me, the sun is shining. To the right, a double rainbow spreads across the sky. The pallbearers come again with their heavy burden and lower it into the grave.

This is the time people usually depart from a burial, leaving the final covering to the gravediggers. But the gravediggers, the pallbearers and the priest are a family of mourners and so we bury her ourselves. Each of the men in turn takes the shovel and casts down the earth: Hugo first, then Jan Barend, then the other men and boys.

Finality is the sound of earth on a coffin, which we usually escape. This time, we wait until it is finished. Some stand quietly, others weep, one woman friend gives a dreadful cry of lament. We draw close in groups and comfort each other. Finally the children gather rocks to put around and mark the grave, the final one a heart-shaped rock found and placed there by 12-year-old Kara.

Deedee and Sandy climb to the highest point of the koppie, just above the grave, to look at Isobel's view. I go over to join them.

'I've already lost two friends in the past 12 months,' I say, 'and now Isobel. It's enough. Don't go anywhere you two. Look after yourselves.'

When we turn round, Hugo has gone, walking back by himself. We drive to the farmhouse, to a long table that has been set up, stretching from one side of the house to the other, through doorways and onto the stoep. We feast and we drink to Isobel.

People remain through the night, with the children sleeping on the flat roof. Peter and I stay at a nearby guest-house and breakfast the next day with an old friend of Isobel's who has come from South Africa. When Hugo comes to see her off, I hug him close once more before we, too, leave for home. He says he will see me the following Friday for breakfast at the Brasilian.

The evening before, I had tried to comfort Hugo. Or was I comforting myself? I am plagued by the questions: How do you do enough for your children? How do you prepare them for your death? I remember Isobel saying to me that she just wanted to stay alive for the children. I need to believe that Jan Barend and Kara will be all right.

'You must know that she has given them everything she can,' I said to Hugo. 'Even though of course she wanted to live longer to be with them, Isobel gave the children all she had. It is there in them; they can draw on it. It will see them through.'

Our Christmas celebration had been in Windhoek, with my parents who were visiting from England. We had merged the Namibian and English Christmas traditions, starting on the evening of the 24th December with a family meal of beef casserole with couscous salad. We continued by putting out stockings for Father Christmas for the children and my parents. On the 25th we opened presents, spent a lazy day together and prepared roast turkey, roast potatoes and vegetables for a meal at 6 p.m. with other family members; it was much too hot to eat such a heavy meal at midday.

Isabel was the only child. Perivi had already left for London, deciding that he must get moving before he drifted. He had packed his life into two large suitcases that were much too heavy to cope with on public transport when he arrived. We tried to persuade him to stay with relatives or family friends but he went to stay with other young Namibians instead.

A few days after Christmas, we drove to Swakopmund and booked into a little hotel right by the sea. It was while we were there that we heard that Isobel had died. I took the call from Deedee while we were looking at gemstones in a little shop.

'I've got bad news,' Deedee said. I had already heard about Isobel's collapse and spoken to her on the phone while she was in hospital, so I knew immediately what it was.

'Oh no. No,' was all I could say. I left the shop and stood on the corner outside.

'We're gathering at Denise's place in Langstrand,' Deedee told me. 'Will you join us?'

'Yes,' I replied, as the tears came.

I went to Langstrand to join Deedee, Sandy and Denise, and their shell-shocked children, sitting on the small stoep that overlooked the ocean, not knowing what to say or do, paralysed by the thought of how suddenly Isobel had gone.

The others returned early to Windhoek because there was no joy anymore in being away on holiday, and because they wanted to be near Hugo and the children. We stayed longer, as we had planned this trip for my parents.

Swakopmund sits at the edge of the desert, a small German town that grew during the colonial period, its small jetty vital to offload goods, soldiers, settlers and unknown mail-order brides from the ships that came from Hamburg and Bremen. The streets are wide, untarred, the surfaces made of hard, impacted, salty sand. It rains no more than 50mm each year but, if it does, the roads become too slippery to drive. The German influence is still strong, with many German-speaking Namibians living there. Shops, and even a few cafés, close for an hour or two at lunchtime. The older buildings in the centre of town are from the early twentieth century, in what is known as 'Kaiser Wilhelm' style. They are two-storied, with high windows and tiled roofs, often with a little circular tower on one corner. The main street was named after Kaiser Wilhelm until recently, when it was changed to Sam Nujoma Avenue.

Most mornings, we woke up to the coastal fog that stretches up to 50 kilometres inland, formed by cold air over the cold sea coming into contact with hot air over the desert; the wind and heat blow it away by lunchtime. The fog also condenses on the desert floor, providing moisture for lichen and small creatures, and creating an eco-system where springbok, oryx and (in the northern Namib Desert) even elephants can survive. The desert itself has many variations – sand dune, gravel plains and mountain ranges – and the colours change from grey to blue, to pink, orange and beige.

Our rooms were on the first floor of the hotel, and my parents climbed the stairs with ease. I was surprised to find them difficult. I had to force my legs to move, holding onto the banister to pull myself up, feeling that I had no strength. I made sure I had what I wanted for the day before I left our room, so I didn't have to face the stairs too many times.

We took my parents on a drive across the undulating, rocky, moon landscape outside Swakopmund, and to see the ancient Welwitschia plants that are over 1000 years old. We walked round town to find a newspaper or pause for morning coffee. We watched the pelicans sitting on the lampposts or hovering where the fishermen cleaned their catch, and went to the small aquarium, where we walked through the Perspex see-through tunnel, looking up at the undersides of shark and sting-rays. Walking along the beach, round rocks where the waves broke dramatically, we bumped into people we knew from Windhoek who were also on holiday, and chatted to them as we strolled along. As we walked back to the hotel, I slowed down. I had no energy and my legs were tired. The others went on ahead, arriving at the hotel long before me.

Later in January, when we are back in Windhoek, after Isobel's funeral, and my parents have returned to the UK, my feet and ankles swell up painfully. I go to the doctor and we decide it's probably the heat – my ankles have swelled up in the past although not this badly. The doctor gives me a diuretic, which helps but does not completely take the problem away. All my shoes have become too tight, so I buy new red sandals that stretch across my fat feet, and begin to prepare in earnest to move out of the shop in a few weeks' time.

Deedee arranges a special breakfast for her 45th birthday in early February. She has booked a table at the mountain-top restaurant of a new hotel. We all plan to be there, but the day before I have a bad headache and feel very weak. I phone Deedee.

'Sorry, Deedee, I'm not going to make it. I'm really not feeling well and I can't face the thought of getting up before seven. I need to lie in a bit.'

I take two days off work again and then struggle to get up and keep going. I'm moving to a tiny office that I'll use as a base for my marketing work. It's right opposite the Brasilian.

We make an effort to continue meeting there as usual on Friday mornings but it's difficult to go back after Isobel's death. The waitresses are glad to see us, but very upset – they knew Isobel well because she was such a regular client. We see Hugo there at times, and he joins us for a while, but of course it is not the same.

As we breakfast there the week after Deedee's birthday, everyone comments on how I look.

'Wow, Jane! You've lost a lot of weight!'

'Yes.'

'You're looking thin!'

'It's the new tight top and skirt,' I say. 'I thought I'd buy something different.' Normally, I wear long, loose, African dresses in bright colours; they are perfect for the Namibian climate.

We talk about our plans for the coming year.

'What about you, Jane?' Deedee asks me. 'What do you want to do?'

'All I want to do is sleep,' I tell them.

I feel exhausted. Walking up the incline to the bank slows me down. Carrying boxes of files or books to my new office is much harder than I expect. I struggle to keep going during the day and lie down as soon as I get home, horizontal on the sofa with my feet up, watching television for an hour. Then I make myself a sandwich and crawl to bed. Peter and Isabel have to get their own evening meal. I wake in the middle of the night, dreaming that I cannot breathe, and sit up to recover. I go to the dining room and sit down. A 1000 piece jigsaw puzzle that my brother and sister-in-law sent out with my parents at Christmas is spread across the table. It's a new take on jigsaws, called a 'Wasgij'. The picture on the box is of a wedding party outside a church, taken from behind the back of the photographer. But the picture formed by the pieces inside is what the bride and groom are looking at, so it's really hard to work out. Doing it focuses my mind on something completely different. After an hour I return to bed and sleep a little more.

'I'm worried about you, Janie,' Deedee tells me. 'You're ill too often. I think you need a real rest, not just a day or two here and there.'

'Give up the marketing work as well,' Sandy urges me. 'You don't need to be doing that. You should be writing.'

Every time we meet, they talk to me about it. Deedee plugs away at me more because she sees me more often – or makes the effort to see me more often in order to talk to me about it. I don't disagree with them but I don't know how to get out of my commitments. I don't enjoy the marketing workshops, though they seem to be a sensible option as they will enable me to continue to work with books and provide a reasonable income.

Deedee pushes all our discussions to the question of my health.

'You should go to the doctor, you know, and find out what's going on. It's not good for you, Jane. And you should tell the publisher that you can't do the marketing after all. It's no big deal. They'll find someone else. Tell them you're going to stop.'

She looks at the calendar and suggests a date when I could say I will stop. Then she pulls it forward bit by bit. She phones or sees me every day.

I tell her of the depression I felt before Christmas, the feeling of defeat I had, the morbidity, playing requiems for myself.

'Talk to the doctor about all that,' she says.

'I would feel foolish telling the doctor that I'm tired,' I reply.

My resistance doesn't last much longer. One weekend, I make the decision not to do the marketing and write the letter to the publishing company. I say simply that I'm exhausted and need to give up all work and rest for six months. I deliver the letter on a Monday in late February to their local publishing manager and also email it to their headquarters so there can be no argument. I'm due to finish clearing out the shop on the Thursday so I make an appointment for Thursday midday with the doctor.

Wednesday is the first anniversary of Brigitte's death. I send a fax to Luther and her parents, remembering her and sending them our love. The next day I finish at the shop and leave it completely empty, except for the painters who are there to get it ready for the next tenant. I depart as a friend loads a bakkie with the last remaining pieces of furniture and a dismantled counter that I had custom-made eight years before. I set off to the doctor, rehearsing in my head what to say, how to explain my exhaustion. All I really want is to go home and sleep but I know that Deedee will tell me off if I don't see the doctor. So it is Deedee who saves my life.

My German GP views health holistically, prescribing natural medicines as first choice, unless your condition clearly needs something different. She prides herself on starting her diagnosis as she watches the way you walk through the door.

'I'm feeling really tired,' I start. 'I keep taking time off but I don't get any better. In fact, I feel so tired I've decided to stop work altogether.'

'By the look of you, I would say that it's something more than tiredness,' she responds.

The moment she examines me, she discovers that my liver is enlarged, the artery in my neck is enlarged, and my pulse is down to 39 instead of a normal 70 or more.

'I think there's a problem with your heart,' she tells me. 'You'll have to go to the hospital for a heart sonar and chest X-ray,' and she phones the physician to arrange for him to meet me there.

'Do you want someone to take you home?'

'No, I'll be alright,' I say. 'I'll phone my husband.'

I drive home in a daze, phone Peter, explain, and ask him to come and take me to the private hospital covered by our medical aid. It's early afternoon and Isabel has just returned from school. I tell her simply that I need to have an X-ray, but Peter makes her come as well.

They whisk me in for a chest X-ray and on to the sonar department. Peter and Isabel sit on hard chairs in the corridor while I go into the small cubicle where the sonar equipment is. I take off my clothes from the waist up and lie down on a hard flat, narrow, bed covered in sheets of green paper. The technician rubs gel on my chest and guides the head of the sonar over my skin, up and down and back again. She turns to the computer and takes measurements across a shadowy image of my heart that's on the screen. As she checks the valves of my heart, the blood shows up red and blue on the computer screen – oxygenated and not oxygenated – pulsing through my heart.

'Heartblock, third degree,' diagnoses the sonar technician. You'll need a pacemaker. You're lucky it isn't viral myocarditis. Then you would need a transplant.'

I don't understand what this means. The first word I recognise is 'pacemaker' but I know nothing about them. The second word I recognise is 'transplant' and there's no way I can deal with that one. I don't know what viral myocarditis is.

I put my clothes back on and go out of the cubicle into the corridor.

'There's something wrong with my heart,' I whisper to Peter. He looks shocked but says nothing.

'I have to go and wait for the doctor,' I tell Isabel. She looks anxious and confused.

An orderly comes to take me up to a ward with four beds. Two of them are already occupied. Peter and Isabel follow me in.

'Just wait on the bed,' the nurse tells me. 'The doctor will be here soon.'

'Do I have to undress and get into bed?' I ask.

'Not right now. We'll see what the doctor says.' She draws pale blue curtains round the bed and I sit on the edge, wondering what's happening.

The physician arrives – the same one under whose care I had the tests at the end of last year. I trust him. He brings my X-ray and sonar results, consults them and looks at the notes at the end of my bed.

'The X-ray shows that your heart is enlarged,' he says. 'The natural pacemaker that controls the heartbeat is not functioning.'

I can see that the notes in his hand say 'heart failure'.

'That sounds a bit strong,' I say.

He looks at me as if I'm rather strange and asks me how I've been feeling.

'I get tired when I'm walking. My ankles have swelled up badly. I feel short of breath at times and I wake up at night feeling I don't have enough air to breathe. I feel so exhausted at the end of the day that I can hardly move.'

'These are all classic symptoms of heart failure,' he tells me, 'caused by the fact that your heart's natural pacemaker isn't functioning. You'll need a pacemaker. I want to take you to ICU now so that we can put you on a heart monitor while we arrange everything.'

I'm taken down the corridor to the Intensive Care Unit. It's stark in comparison with the previous ward. One other patient is there, horizontal and silent. The walls and curtains are white. Machines stand along the wall. The nurses plug the electrodes of an ECG machine onto my chest and ankles and connect me. I can see the pattern of my heartbeat on the screen and the number flashing in green that counts the number of beats per minute. Peter and Isabel hover by my bed. We are all in shock. I thought I would be given some pills and sent home to rest. None of us expected this.

The doctors decide to send me to Cape Town to see a cardiologist and have the pacemaker fitted there. First they must get approval from the medical aid to pay for it. They scurry round to make the necessary calls and the medical aid company sends another doctor to assess me before giving the go-ahead. My physician recommends that I go as a walking patient with a paramedic.

'If I send you in med-evac,' he says, 'I'll have to sedate you and it's not pleasant.'

I give myself up to the process, placing myself in the hands of the medical personnel who have taken control of my life. I stay in hospital overnight, sleeping sporadically, listening to the beep of the monitor and trying to find a position that's comfortable with all the ECG wires attached to me. In the morning, Peter and Isabel come to see me before I leave. Peter has brought an overnight bag with toiletries and a nightie, for me to take with me.

'We couldn't get on the same flight,' he tells me, rubbing my feet gently. 'But we're on the one afterwards. So we'll be there with you.'

'Isabel as well?' I ask.

'Yes, Mummy.' She lies down beside me on the bed. Peter has explained to her what's happening.

'I love you so much, Mummy,' she says.

'I love you too my darling,' I tell her.

'I love you more.'

There's not much I can say to comfort her so we hold onto each other until it's time for me to go.

A paramedic arrives to accompany me to Cape Town. I'm unplugged from all the wires and I get dressed, putting on loose trousers and a shirt. The paramedic takes me in a wheelchair to the hospital door. Peter and Isabel are left there while I get into a medical rescue car that takes me to the airport. I walk slowly to the head of the check-in queue, through passport control, and sit down in the departure lounge. The paramedic has a bag of medical equipment that sets off all the security scanners. He checks my blood pressure and pulse during the flight, while the other passengers peer at us to see what's going on. When we arrive in Cape Town, we are picked up by an ambulance and taken to the Panorama Clinic on the northern side of Table Bay.

Twenty-four hours after seeing my GP in Windhoek, I'm in Cape Town in the same Cardiac Special Care Unit from which Isobel was discharged six weeks earlier, on the day of her death. I'm wired up to a heart monitor again and lie on my back in the bed, which is tilted up at the head to lift me a little and help me breathe more easily. When I want to go to the toilet, I have to call the nurse, who comes to unplug me and escort me across the ward. Around the walls are large laminated posters showing diagrams of the heart, highlighting different diseases or problems. I walk slowly round on my way back from the toilet, before being plugged back onto the monitors. I look at the posters, trying to make sense of what has happened to me and what happened to Isobel. One of the nurses comes to reconnect me to the monitor, and I ask,

'Do you remember a woman from Namibia who was here just after Christmas? She had a massive heart attack. Her name was Isobel.'

'Yes,' replies the nurse. 'I remember her. I don't think she knew just how ill she was.'

'What happened?' I ask.

'Well, as I remember it, she had been on a portable monitor, so we were checking her heart from up here even when she was out of the ward. She seemed to be recovering. But the day she went down to the doctor's rooms they removed the monitor, because she was going to go home. Maybe we could have seen something happening if the monitor had still been on, but maybe not. There was a lot of damage from the heart attack, and her heart just didn't make it.'

I discover that the cardiologist who admits me is the same doctor who had seen Isobel, but I don't want to ask him anything more about what happened to her.

Peter and Isabel come in the next morning to see me. They stay in a small bed and breakfast right next to the hospital, which is often used by Namibian families visiting patients here.

The doctor to whom I've been consigned is off duty for the weekend, so I end up having to wait for a Monday appointment with technology. I sleep on and off throughout the next two days and nights. I watch my heartbeat tick away on the monitor, slowing down all the time. By Sunday night the number of beats per minute is below 30 – less than half what it should be. I have no energy at all and I'm grateful just to be horizontal. I still can't take in what is happening to me but there's nothing I can do; my fate is in the hands of others.

The ward is circular, with the nurses' station in the middle. Most of the patients are attached to heart monitors and there is a buzz of noise from the machines but no conversation between the patients – the beds are too far apart. Close family visitors are allowed, and phone calls. I get many. Peter has told Perivi and my parents what's happening and they call me, including my younger sister Helen, who is living in Mexico.

I don't know when they invented pacemakers, but I thank whoever did. It doesn't require an operation, just a 'procedure', because it is done with local anaesthetic. The insertion of this matchbox-sized battery doesn't take long. A 3cm incision is made on one side of my chest; a tiny electrode is threaded through a vein right into the heart; the pacemaker is tucked under the skin, tested, and switched on. I live.

My heart is 'set' at 70 beats per minute. I must remain in the hospital for three days, while they monitor my progress. On the second day, while I'm dozing, the nurse brings the phone to me. It's Doris.

'What's this, my dear?' she asks me. 'What's going on?'

'I don't know,' I say. 'I don't know what's happening to me. Where are you? Can you come and see me?'

The next day, Doris drives over to see me. I've been moved into a different ward. My condition is improving but the nurses are still checking my heartbeat through a monitor that hangs round my neck, with five electrodes attached across my chest. It's much easier for me to move about, and to find a comfortable position in which to sleep.

'Come over to the window,' Doris says. 'There's something I want you to see.'

The window looks across Table Bay. The day is clear and there's a magnificent view of Table Mountain, with no cloud covering the top.

'Wow,' I say. 'That's the second best view of Table Mountain I've ever had.'

'And the best?' Doris asks me.

'From Robben Island, when we went there with Perivi and Isabel two years ago.' We had unexpectedly bumped into Ben Ulenga at the dock in Cape Town, waiting for the boat to Robben Island. He was taking his children to see where he had been imprisoned. But the former prison had been cleaned and decorated and held little sense for me of the terrible place it had once been.

Two days later, we fly back to Windhoek. I move slowly and deliberately but I'm already feeling less tired. I wait a week before phoning Hugo.

'I'm sorry,' I say. 'I was there in the same ward where Isobel was. I saw the same doctor. I thought about her so much. I talked to the nurses about her and they remember her. It was such a good place. The care was good. I'm sure they must have done everything they could have done for Isobel. But I'm sorry. I don't know why I should come home and she didn't...'

'No...' He pauses. 'I know they did what they could. I don't have any problems with them or any worries about that... Thank you for phoning. It should have been me phoning to see how you are.'

'I'm getting stronger,' is all I can say.

'Do nothing for six months,' the doctors told me, 'to give your heart time to recover. Don't walk up any hills. Don't carry anything heavy.'

The whole process has been so quick that I can't react to it. The shock comes slowly afterwards. The collapse of my heart was triggered, the doctors believe, by a viral infection that interrupted the normal electric charge of the heart, causing my pulse to progressively slow down. If I had gone home from the bookshop and taken to my bed, instead of going to the doctor, perhaps I would have never got up again.

An old friend from England hears about my illness and phones:

'Don't be surprised if you feel depressed,' she says. 'Apparently depression often sets in after heart disease or heart problems.'

But I feel not depression so much as sweeping fear. Although I was ill at various times last year, there is no particular episode that stands out as the one that caused my heart to fail. The symptoms developed over a period of months, not suddenly. Looking back, I remember the pain across my chest one night. I remember my heart banging against the mattress when I turned onto my left side at night. Was it already enlarged and failing then, I wonder?

Even though I'm doing nothing now, I still feel dizzy with tiredness at times and have to lie down. I fear that the dizziness is a sign of ongoing infection. I fear that the virus is still in my system and will continue to eat away at my heart. I fear falling asleep and never waking again. I curl up at night in Peter's arms, praying that I will live to see the next day.

111

I talk a lot to Isobel, and to Brigitte. They are my companions. I come to know that the dividing line between life and death is tenuous and insubstantial.

I look for the letter we received a year ago, in the days after Brigitte's death, faxed to the bookshop by Luther, with a message from him asking what we thought of it. It was in German, so I had left it on the desk for Doris, with a note asking her to translate it for me. She came in the next day with translation in hand. She lit a cigarette and looked at me.

'Who and where did this come from?' she asked.

'From Luther. He said something about it coming from Brigitte's cousin. What does it say?'

'Well,' she says, 'I discussed it with Clive and we don't know quite what to make of it.' She showed me the translation (with alternatives for certain words in brackets):

I am well. The journey to the other side is accompanied (complete). Yi-Jiun's spirit guide allows me to write this letter to you through her. This contact is very rare. When someone dies, (s)he dies, no more a word, no further message. I regret that and find it sad, that one can no longer speak to each other. My illness weighed heavily on me, in this recent time. I thank you from the bottom of my heart, for all you have done for me. There were times when I did not give up so quickly because of your caring. But the time has come. I have completed this life. I have done what I had planned and now the time has come to take a break, to take some rest. You must not worry about me, but care for yourselves as well as possible. Mutti and Vati are already old. Maybe they will someday themselves have to come to terms with the subject of death. I will wait for them with open arms and welcome them. Here everything is very beautiful. I, for the first time know why I am born on earth – simply to experience all that there is not here.
I will not tell you too much now. I wish you happiness (luck) for the rest of your lives on earth. Be grateful, that you could be human (grow as men). That is like a gift!

Adieu, Brigitte

After reading the letter, I had phoned Luther immediately to try to find out what it was. He explained that he had received it the night that Brigitte died, from her cousin, who had not yet been informed of her death. The cousin received the message as an email from a former girlfriend of his, Yi-Jiun, who had a reputation as a medium.

I thought long and hard about it. I discussed it with Doris, with Peter and again with Luther. There was no way round it, I felt. It must be a weird stunt or a communication from a dimension beyond this life.

'It's like a dream from the ancestors,' Peter said.

I thought it sounded compellingly like Brigitte's voice and it led me to accept that her spirit continued to exist on some other plane.

I needed to share this with the others and the best time to get them all together was in the bustle of Friday breakfast at the Brasilian.

'I want to tell you about something extraordinary. It's to do with Brigitte. You all stood by me when I was so upset at her death, so I want you to see this.'

I explained how it came to me and passed it round to them. Isobel was the most struck by it.

'I knew it,' she said.

A month after my hospitalisation, in late March 2003, US and UK government forces invade Iraq. It is the final step in a long build up of threats and the first step in a terrible war. Journalists 'embedded' with their troops send frontline news and views to households all over the world. My mind rejects the reasons for troops being there and in my current state my every cell is appalled. I can't watch or listen to the news, dominated as it is by the war.

Films that I would ordinarily enjoy are rendered violent by my vulnerability. Favourite detective stories are out – even those that don't show any blood. I can't deal with intense emotions or intense discussions. My heart literally hurts.

I wake late, bathe slowly, dress sometimes and sleep a lot. I rest in bed every afternoon listening to classical music. I cannot yet read.

'Reading has always been such an important part of my life,' I say to Peter. 'Now I can't concentrate and I'm not even interested.'

I abandon any role within the family. Peter gets Isabel up in the morning and off to school. He organises transport for her after-school activities. He does the shopping. Other friends help with that too. Our housekeeper Alexia does the cooking and cleaning. She has looked after us since we came to Namibia, helping to raise the children and enabling me to pursue my own career. She makes me feel safe while I am resting. I can hear her pottering around, answering the phone and taking messages so that I can continue to rest. I can hear her managing my home while I sleep or rest, or play card games on the computer for the first time in my life – it's mindless and it passes the time.

I lie in my bed looking at the garden and the jacaranda tree outside my window. I sit in the lounge looking at the view over Windhoek. I sit in the courtyard listening to the birds. I listen to music. It's too much effort to do anything else. Even sitting for too long makes me tired.

The only effort I make is to see my GP. She has told me that she wants to see me regularly so she can monitor my progress. I ask her one question that worries me:

'How will I die, if my heart is being kept going by this battery? I have this surreal image of being buried with my heart still beating away but all the rest of me – my organs, brain, everything – dead.'

'Don't worry,' she replies. 'You can die.'

I am aided in my convalescence by Mosé's wife Sandra, to whom I've always felt very close. When I first came to Namibia I had hoped I would spend more time with her, but she already had a circle of close friends who had been together with her in Lusaka – a group of African and African-American women. I felt very aware of my Englishness when I was with them. Sandra was also busy accompanying Mosé to official dinners and on official trips that are part of his work.

Sandra, too, has had heart problems, and has a pacemaker. I've never asked her much about it. Now we sit in our courtyard and she advises me.

'They put it in and send you off and never tell you how to cope with it,' she says. 'But your whole body will be fighting against it for months. Think about it. There is this foreign object inserted into your body. It is metallic. It is electric. It sends an electric impulse down your veins and right into your heart. It is going to take some time for you to get used to that, so don't expect too much of yourself.'

She pauses. 'I did too much after my pacemaker was inserted. I travelled to the US. I tried to keep going and I ended up back in hospital with liver problems. If you don't give your heart the time to recover, your other organs will try to compensate and they will suffer.'

'After that, I stopped,' she continues. 'I really slowed down. I remember all I watched on television was National Geographic. I used to see the animals, the wildlife, on those programmes, and say to myself: "They are alive. I am alive."'

'I'm just so frightened,' I reply. 'The scar where they inserted the pacemaker aches. My heartbeat seems to bounce sometimes. I feel exhausted. I feel useless. I don't know what I'm supposed to do or not do.'

'No, my dear,' she says. 'You know what you have been told to do. You have been told to do nothing for six months. So you do nothing for six months. Just be. Your children need you to be there. Your children need you to continue to be there for them. Just hold on to that. You don't have to work. You don't have to achieve anything. Just be.'

Two years ago, after an operation, I didn't drive for three weeks and it seemed such a long time. Now I decide that I'm not going to drive for three months, so that I won't get sucked into doing too much. I get lifts to the doctor's – mostly it is Deedee who takes me. I get lifts to the café if we meet for coffee. Friends collect me to take me to their houses.

Gradually, as I start to go out a bit more, I get lifts to the supermarket and walk slowly round choosing fruit or bread and letting someone else carry them.

Perivi comes home for a month from London. He looks thinner than when he left and his hair is longer than he's ever had it before, brushed into an Afro style. I haven't seen him since before my pacemaker was inserted, although I've talked to him on the phone, and I rejoice to have him home again. My illness and his distance have swept away the tension that had grown between us because of conflicts over his late nights. He tells me about his life in London – he has been working as a night security guard at exhibition centres, a quiet job that gives him time to read.

My parents come once more. They are in their eighties now but they are fit and energetic, living independently and looking after themselves in the farmhouse that belonged to my grandparents, where my grandfather and uncle farmed. Their pace is faster than mine. They walk down to the shops to buy bread and back up the steep hill again. My father drives me to the doctor. They sit with me and read while I rest.

My brother John comes to be with me for a few days after a conference in South Africa. He is an Anglican minister in London and leads a charismatic renewal movement that emphasises personal experience of the Spirit of God, and the power of healing, prophesying and speaking in tongues. He stays in Perivi's flat after Perivi has returned to London, and uses the quiet time to also to finish a booklet he is writing, on healing.

I am surrounded by love.

Talking to my GP one day, I ask her why this happened to me.

'You fell off the mountain,' she says.

The image stays with me and I go back to the house and ponder on it. I need to try to define what has happened; maybe then I can move beyond it. Reflecting through the day and in my waking moments, words come to me and bit by bit I write out my life's journey:

> Long ago, when I was small, I lived in a green valley, surrounded by family and by love. But I could see that there were other worlds outside our valley. I could see that there was suffering out there. And I could see that there was more

116

beauty even than in our valley. I longed for sharper, clearer air.

So I set off on my journey and I came to the foothills of the mountain that is Life and I started to climb.

There were friends along the way who made their own decisions about where to settle. But I moved on.

I came across a companion who inspired me to climb with him, to see the beauty, to challenge the suffering, to breathe the pure air higher up the mountain. So we climbed together. He was much stronger than me, and more agile. He ran ahead and ran back to report to me and to rest his head on my lap. I climbed more slowly, pausing to contemplate and to take time to look around me.

We climbed for many years. There were difficult times, when we scrambled over obstacles and clung to one another. There were good times, when we felt we were soaring. There were times when the mountain was shrouded in mist and we could not see where we were going. And there were times when we had to concentrate just on putting one foot in front of the other in order to keep moving.

Over the years, we gathered children – our own and others' – and loved them and tried to lead them to their own paths. But anxieties about their safety took their toll. The fear of them losing their footholds was hard.

And over the years, we took on many other burdens – responsibilities for this project and for that project. We felt that so much needed to be done, so we tried to do it all. My companion rushed on ahead, and I forgot to stop and look around me, barely pausing as I tried to keep pace.

Higher up the mountain, the air grew thinner and it became harder to breathe. The rocks were sharper. The paths were steeper. We walked on a knife-edge, precariously balancing all our loads, bending down to keep going against the wind, so that we rarely saw the beautiful views.

I came to understand that I needed to climb more slowly. I started to let go of some of my load. I looked for a place to stop, or a path that would be easier. But in trying to prepare a new way, I took on more responsibilities again – and my heart was not in it.

I thought I could make one last effort and get to some sort of haven. But I was too tired from all my years of climbing. I lost my footing and fell.

I fell down, down, down, to the bottom of the mountain, to a place of shadows and fear. Broken and bruised. My loved ones caught me and held me close. Medical science patched me up so that I could move again. I sit, waiting for the bruises to heal, knowing that I cannot climb anymore and that a new path will reveal itself to me.

'Part of your recovery will be to accept that you have recovered and to give thanks,' my GP tells me. So I go to church, for the first time in many months, to St George's, the tiny Anglican cathedral in Windhoek. Made out of old yellowed sandstone, with a bell outside but no tower or spire, it seats less than 200 people.

I was raised and confirmed in the Anglican Church in Leeds, but when I went to university I learned what had been done in colonial times in the name of Christianity, and how the established churches had supported and endorsed conquest and injustice. I stopped going to church and became involved in politics.

'When the missionaries came to Africa they had the Bible and we had the land,' South African Archbishop Desmond Tutu has joked. 'They said, "Let us pray." We closed our eyes. When we opened them we had the Bible and they had the land.'

In my work on Southern Africa in the 1970s, however, I came into contact with churchmen and women like Archbishop Tutu, who actively campaigned for an end to apartheid and injustice in South Africa and Namibia. These included Bishop Colin Winter, who had introduced me to Peter.

Colin Winter was a British priest who had himself experienced inequality as a child growing up in a poor family in England. After being ordained, he worked for six years in South Africa, before moving to become Dean of St George's in Windhoek, in 1964. Four years later, the South African authorities deported the Anglican Bishop, Robert Mize, and Colin Winter took over as Bishop and head of the Anglican Church in Namibia.

Most churches in Namibia grew out of the German and Finnish Lutheran missionary work that started in the mid-nineteenth century. The Anglican Church came late to the country. It's a small community of believers, with congregations concentrated in Walvis Bay, Windhoek and along the Namibia/Angola border in the Ohangwena region.

Passionate about Namibia and its people, and actively involved in the cause of Namibia's freedom, Bishop Winter was deported from the country by the South Africans in 1972. He believed thereafter that he, too, was in exile. He had a series of heart attacks but he threw himself into campaigning in Britain and internationally for the cause of Namibian freedom.

'The gospel challenges society, and is, above all, about liberation,' he preached. 'Being faithful to the gospel means challenging society.' He wanted the church to break with its historic past and side with the poor.

Bishop Winter challenged the South African authorities in Namibia and denounced imprisonment and torture under South African rule. He challenged the establishment of the Church of England in Britain that had investments in South Africa. When there was conflict within SWAPO in 1976 and eleven dissidents were imprisoned in Zambia, without charge or trial, he also challenged the SWAPO leadership about this. I began to see that Bishop Winter and others like him were the ones to witness consistently on issues of human rights. When he died in 1981, I told myself at his funeral that I would give his faith another chance.

We were living in Oxford then and I went occasionally to what had been Bishop Winter's church in Oxford after he was expelled from Namibia. We baptised Perivi there when he was two, choosing one set of godparents from Namibia and another from England. His English godmother, Margaret, had worked closely with Bishop Winter. His Namibian godfather, Daniel, was a SWAPO leader inside Namibia and a top official of the Council of Churches in Namibia. On one of his trips, Peter had bought Perivi a little West African suit – cotton trousers and loose shirt in beige and soft browns, with gold embroidery down the front of the shirt. Perivi wore it at his baptism; I wore an African dress I had that was in the same colours.

I joined a women's group in Oxford that met each month to discuss Christianity. I went to the United Church of Christ at Yale University, when we were in America. I loved the woman priest in charge there, and the liturgy – a combination of silence and song. Isabel was baptised there when she was ten months old and we were able to write some of our own words for her blessing.

Again, I had matching outfits for Isabel and me. I wore a light blue African dress and there was just enough material in the cloth that was supposed to be used as a scarf round my head to make a tiny dress for Isabel. I sewed it by hand.

After Independence, Bishop Winter's ashes were brought to Namibia and placed in an urn in the walls of St George's cathedral. I have worshipped there occasionally but not regularly. I found the services slow and the hymns difficult.

However, since I was rushed to hospital in Cape Town, my name has been added to the list of those in need of healing, on the service sheet at St George's. People have been praying for me there.

'How are you, Jane?' they ask when I go there one Sunday morning.

'Are you recovering?'

'You look too thin.'

'Is there anything we can do to help?'

I don't know how much they know about what's happened to me but their concern warms me. I decide that I will go to church again and stand up to say thank you for their prayers and thank you to God for bringing me through this.

Feeling more confident, I get up earlier and see Isabel off to school. I take my place once more as mother and carer. I start to drive. I pop out to pick up food from the shops, to drop Isabel at her after-school activities or pick her up.

Isabel's work has not been going well with all the disruption and distress caused by my being ill. She's found it difficult to concentrate since I was in hospital and we came back from Cape Town. She also complains to me about two of her teachers.

'One of them is just so boring. I don't see any point in being in her lessons. I'm not learning anything. She doesn't seem to know what she's talking about. It's awful.

'The other one has given us two weeks to do a science project. But she hasn't said what she really wants us to do. I don't know how long it must be. I don't know what sort of project it should be. She doesn't seem really interested.'

Isabel starts to work on the project with a friend who comes round to our house. They spend the afternoon discussing it and decide they will do something on HIV/AIDS. They spend more afternoons researching on the internet. I ask Jane for help with materials and she brings some to breakfast that Friday. Isabel and her friend decide to visit one of the New Start centres where people can go for counselling and voluntary testing for HIV/AIDS, to interview the staff. She phones to make the necessary appointment but she still feels unsure about what they're supposed to be doing.

'I'm going to get in touch with the school as well,' I tell Isabel. 'They should guide you better you in something like this.' I write to explain my concerns and request a meeting. I'm given an appointment for three days later, with two senior teachers.

'We've discussed your letter with Isabel's teachers, particularly the teachers of those subjects you refer to,' they tell me when we meet. 'The teachers feel that Isabel is not putting enough into her work and that the problem is her attitude.'

A wave of anger at this stock reply overwhelms me. I take a deep breath and try to stay calm.

'First of all,' I say, 'I think you know I've been seriously ill. It's not been easy for Isabel. But apart from that, I feel you should listen to what she's saying.' I turn to one particular teacher. 'For instance, you've taught Perivi and Isabel and they've both said what a good teacher you are. Everyone listens to children when they say a teacher is good. Their assessment is taken seriously.' I pause. 'Why is their assessment not taken seriously if they feel a teacher is not very good?'

My heart beats fast. I try to argue but I feel physically weak. My confidence evaporates.

The following week, after coffee with a friend in town, I feel exhausted. I go home and sleep for three hours in the afternoon and another ten hours that night. Sleep helps but there is a changed rhythm to my heartbeat. It gives little extra beats and sometimes my whole chest seems to jump. Does this mean that my heart is degenerating further? I wonder. Am I going to die? What then will happen to Isabel?

My GP sees me floundering. 'It doesn't matter if you are trying to swim and can't do it properly, the pacemaker is like a swimming ring, keeping you afloat, and it's attached to a boat by a line,' she tells me. She does an ECG. The pulse of the pacemaker looks good but we see an irregular heartbeat coming unevenly every now and then.

She phones my physician to get it checked. He sends me for another chest X-ray and heart sonar. Peter is away, so Deedee takes me to the small Catholic hospital, even though she arrived home this morning after a trip to see her parents in the USA. We wait at the hospital for the physician. I'm shown into an area of cubicled beds with curtains drawn round them, which provide little privacy, however, because you can hear everything that other patients are discussing with their doctors. Deedee sits on the end of the bed and chats quietly about her holiday. I don't hear what she says.

'Sorry, Deedee. I'm not really with it. I just want the doctor to come,' I tell her.

My physician arrives, hooks me up to the ECG and checks the one that had been done earlier by my GP. He checks the results of the heart sonar and chest X-ray.

'Well, your heart is not enlarged anymore,' he says. 'That's good news. The function of the heart is reduced a bit, but not enough to worry about. What you have is an extra heartbeat that comes and goes. We can give you some medication for that. It's not really an arrhythmia. It's maybe one part of the heart that is doing its own thing, beating from time to time. You have what we call an "undisciplined heart".'

My undisciplined heart. It started when I was pregnant with Perivi – an irregular beat to my heart that continued through the pregnancy, forcing me to give up coffee and tea in an age when there were virtually no decaffeinated variants available. The doctors told me it was a response to the changing hormones.

It beat irregularly when I was ill or feverish and last year, after I came home from saying goodbye to Brigitte. It bumped at night uncomfortably when my heart became enlarged. It slowed down to next-to-nothing at the beginning of the year. An electronic device now paces it. I must accept the balance this gives me and not fight against it.

The beating of a heart, like the beating of a drum, and the march of time. Beating when I first met the man who became my husband. Beating in love, beating in pain, beating in sickness, beating now to keep me going.

My undisciplined heart, taking me far away from the comfort of known English shores and a safe existence, to the liberation struggle of Southern Africa.

On Isobel's birthday we gather for a special breakfast at the Brasilian – Deedee, Sandy, me, Isobel's sister, Hugo, and his mother who is visiting. Jane is away at an international AIDS conference. It's a sad occasion but good for us to be able to remember Isobel this day. Since Isobel's death, her sister has made big changes in her life. She has found a new job and left her husband, deciding that life is short and there was no point staying in a marriage that had already failed.

Perhaps prompted by Isobel's death at the age of 47, and my heart failure, Sandy has started to look at ways to take more care of herself. She gives up smoking, again, and this time she is sure she will succeed. She also decides to have an old mole cut out of her thigh.

'I've had it for years,' she explains. 'It looks dark but it hasn't changed in appearance, which is what they say you must look out for. Anyway, I want to have it removed.'

She talks to her GP, who thinks it isn't necessary but, at her insistence, he books her in to see the specialist.

As a matter of course, they do a biopsy on the mole after cutting it out and they find melanoma cells – one of the most virulent and dangerous types of cancer. They inform Sandy by telephone, leaving a message on her answer-phone.

'I came home one day to an empty house – everyone was out – and switched on the answer machine. There was this bloody message telling me I've got cancer, and telling me they had already booked me in for it to be cut out!'

A few days later, under local anaesthetic, they cut a long strip of flesh, about a centimetre deep, out of her thigh.

'Honestly, I kid you not,' she says. 'I looked down at the wrong time and saw the flesh they had cut away. I saw the blood running down my leg but I couldn't feel anything. Then they bandaged me up and sent me home.'

To find out if the cancer has spread, they do chest and liver X-rays and a CT scan of her kidneys. I wake in the night worrying about her. Cancer is in her family.

A week later Sandy has her third cut, to extract the lymph node at the top of the affected leg. The doctors are still looking to see if the cancer has spread, then they will decide on her treatment.

Jane and I go to see Sandy at home as she recovers. It's my first attempt to climb steep stairs – her house is perched on one of the hills of

Windhoek – but I think I can do it since her father and mother manage the stairs whenever they are visiting, and they are not strong. We drink coffee at her house, abandoning the public space of the Brasilian.

'What's happening to us all?' I ask. 'Why are we collapsing one after the other so suddenly and in such quick succession?'

'I don't know,' Jane says. 'I'm also wondering.' We don't have any answers.

After many tests, the doctors tell Sandy that they think they have cut out all the cancer cells and she doesn't require further treatment, but she must go for regular check-ups to make sure it stays that way.

Home again from teaching abroad, Tricia brings her wry sense of humour to cheer up Sandy. She has been through cancer and reconstructive surgery, so she understands, and she's lived to tell the tale.

'Look at me,' she says. 'Look at what they've done to me and I've survived! If I can survive, then you can too.'

Tricia did not stay long in Scotland. We ask her why.

'Everything was so delayed that I couldn't get a job by the time the school year started. They have to vet you now under new regulations designed to keep sex offenders out of schools. It takes ages.'

'Besides,' she adds. 'As it turned out, my mother didn't need me as much as I thought. She has things well sorted out and my brother helps a lot. So it was really me thinking that I ought to be helping her, rather than the other way round.

'I found a teaching post at an international school in Copenhagen and I took that. I had a flat just near the school, and I cycled everywhere. I would have happily stayed on, except it was only a short-term contract.'

On holiday in Windhoek now, not in school, Tricia is drawn into our Friday breakfasts. She invites us to wonderful lunches at her and Richard's home as well, where we sit long into the afternoon, chatting. However, she has been offered another job at a newly established international school in Luanda and will not be with us for long. She is excited but fearful about going. She hopes it will be like Zambia used to be but she is worried about being alone in a new country and now wishes she could stay in Namibia.

'I'm a wee bit worried about the principal,' she says. 'I've been reading the information for teachers. We're given very specific instructions about what we are allowed to do and not allowed to do. Only single teachers are recruited. No families allowed. No visitors of the opposite gender. And a very strict dress code – definitely no denim. Makes me want to pack denim skirts just to be awkward!'

We give her a red-table send-off at the Brasilian. We have brought flowers, champagne, and a farewell present from us all, chosen by Sandy. Tricia opens it, lets out a shriek of delight and waves it aloft. It is a denim bag embroidered in gold thread.

At breakfast one Friday, Bente announces that she and her family might also be on the move.

'I got a phone call from the council in Arendal,' she tells us. 'They want me to apply for the job as principal of a newly combined primary and secondary school.'

'Bente! You can't go!' Jane says.

'Well, I don't want to,' she replies. 'It's so good being here. The family is so settled. I thought I could ask to stay on another year as well, after my contract finishes. But it won't last forever. Now I don't know what to do.'

'Well, if you do apply, it'll give you time to think about it,' I say. 'But we don't want to lose you.'

Bente discusses it with Uazuvara and their two girls, Ida and Nora. They were reluctant to come to Namibia 18 months ago but now they don't want to leave. Uazuvara has found his place as a philosopher at the cafés and meeting rooms of the town. He has started to write about his grandmother, a survivor of the German massacres, who played a huge role in his childhood and upbringing, and who taught him to accept all people and not hate because of race or tribe. But they must go where Bente has work. She applies for the job and is offered it.

'It'll give us a secure income while the girls grow up and finish their education,' she rationalises, 'and I can be near my parents as they grow older.'

We gather at Deedee's for a farewell dinner for Bente and Uazuvara. For the first time, we bring our husbands. Michael, Hugo and Sandy's husband Ted already know each other well, their sons play cricket together, and the families have all been on outings and holidays together. Peter and Uazuvara are old friends and have come to know Helao since his release from Robben Island. The three of them share the common tradition of the struggle, but not a common experience of it, since Helao was imprisoned while they were in exile.

Peter and Helao start to talk about their different experiences, the early days of SWAPO and the Terrorism Trial, the launch of the armed struggle and one of the guerrilla leaders, who people believe betrayed his comrades to the South Africans.

'I was a conscript in the South African army here,' Hugo tells us. 'Young and confused. I didn't know what I was doing.'

'Where were you?' we ask.

'At Oshivelo.' It is the border point between central Namibia and the northern homeland of Ovamboland, where SWAPO fighters mostly operated.

'He was lucky he wasn't further north, in the thick of things,' I say to Peter later.

Ted also served as a conscript, in the Rhodesian armed forces. Sandy says he hadn't talked about his experiences until he read *Mukiwa*, Peter Godwin's book about growing up in Rhodesia as a young white boy/man. That made him tell Sandy what it had been like. He also talked to their children after one of their friends said he wanted to join the British army, thinking that it would make him tough, a man.

'Make no mistake,' Ted said. 'If you go into the army they will train you to kill people, and you will never be the same again.'

I go to Bente and Uazuvara's house to say goodbye but they are inundated with people calling, in person and on the phone. I go again the morning they leave. As they get into the kombi to go to the airport, relatives of Uazuvara's are still arriving; some take the opportunity to ask for last-minute financial assistance before they go.

I want to tell Bente how good it has been to have their family close to us in Namibia, how good it has been to have her in our Friday breakfast group, how much I have enjoyed having her here. But in her last few days, she is so busy and so much in demand, trying to finish packing for them to leave, that it isn't possible to find a moment when I can say much. So I part from Bente in the middle of a conversation, both literally and figuratively, hoping that it will continue, via email and visits and letters and telepathy. I'm sure that I will see Bente and her family again, in Europe or in Namibia, but it's another step in our group falling apart.

A new branch of the Brasilian has opened in Maerua Mall, the suburban shopping centre on our side of town. The manager has moved across and left the original one in the hands of the practised staff. The menu of the new one is the same but the ambience is different. The shop is large and open, with brown leather sofas and a low table in the centre, square wood tables and chairs, large back-lit murals painted by a young local artist on the walls that depict musicians and people dancing. The clientele is also different – fewer business people and more women shoppers.

During coffee there one morning with Deedee and Sandy, I receive a call from Peter that will change our lives.

'I've just come from State House,' he says.

I imagine discussions about the university because the President is Chancellor, but I am wrong.

'We were talking about my next step after the university.' He pauses. 'The President is appointing me as an ambassador.' Another pause. 'We're supposed to go in a couple of months.'

I'm astounded, and silent. I can't respond out loud in case I give something away. I need to talk to him first to find out more. I get up and walk outside the café.

'Where?' is all I can ask.

'Brussels,' he replies.

This prospect, of an ambassadorial posting after Peter's contract at the university was due to end, was raised last year but I had put it out of my mind. It was impossible to take it into consideration because it was only a suggestion for the future. He has one year of his contract left but that is immediately irrelevant. You do not say 'Wait' to such an appointment.

It is too big to hold in my head, so I hang up and go back to the table. The others are deep in conversation. I drink my decaffeinated cappuccino and keep quiet. I try not to show in my face or physical reactions that something so significant has happened.

Later in the day, when we are face to face at home, Peter confirms it all. I wonder how on earth we will deal with this. We have no fixed date to go and must keep quiet about it until a formal announcement is made.

I worry about myself and whether or not I have the strength to do this. I worry about schools, the best time to go from Isabel's point of view, and when to tell her about it. The Windhoek grapevine takes care of that, though. She comes home from school one day and confronts me.

'Something really odd happened today. A friend told me that her father says we are moving to Sweden.'

It is close enough to the truth for me to come clean.

'Well, we're not moving to Sweden.' It is my turn to pause. 'But we will be moving. The President has appointed Daddy to be ambassador to Brussels. It's all just happened and I don't know more than that. I was going to tell you when I had more details.'

'You're not serious!' she cries. 'This is my home, my Namibia! This is where my friends are! I'm not going!' Then as the thought occurs to her: 'You can leave me here with Uanaingi!'

'I don't think so.'

Although we're not supposed to spread the news, it's impossible to keep it to ourselves. I ask Isabel not to speak about it but she tells her two closest friends.

'I need their help,' she says.

Deedee comes round to see me. Although it's months away, her mind is moving to the end of the year and she wants to start planning.

'What are you doing at Christmas, Jane? Shall we do something together as families?'

I look at her and I can't dissemble.

'We won't be here...' I say and tell her the news.

'Oh Jane,' she says. 'We're going to miss you.'

Later, drinking tea on Deedee's balcony, I tell Sandy and Jane.

'Jane-Jane,' Sandy says. 'It's nice for you but not so nice for us.'

We phone Perivi in London to give him the news; he is excited. He comes back to help prepare for our departure and decides it's time to plan his own his next move. He takes up the offer of a place to study in the USA in a college that has a link to the University of Namibia.

I try to be positive; to look forward to the move as a new beginning for me, but at times it seems like another mountain that needs climbing. I feel as if I'm on a plateau and have no strength to climb any further. If you pick me up and move me, I might be all right, but I don't know if I can get there by myself.

On bad days what I fear most is that I will get to Europe and die soon thereafter. What will happen to Isabel then, uprooted from her life, without a mother? What will I do without Deedee if I fall ill when Peter is away?

Peter's name must be submitted and approved by the three kingdoms to which he will be accredited – Belgium, Luxembourg and The Netherlands, as well as by the European Union. Until that is done, no official announcement can be made. Progress is slow. Peter must prepare to hand over at the university, so he is preoccupied with that. I research schools in Brussels and make initial enquiries about a place for Isabel. There is a British school and an International School that interest me.

At lunch one day at Tricia's, we sit in the garden and I tell them about the schools. By now, all my friends know about our imminent departure.

'What do you think? Which would be better for Isabel?' I ask them.

'How would they follow on from what Isabel's doing now?' asks Tricia.

'The British School does GCSE, which is close to what she would do here, then A-levels.' I reply. 'Peter suggests the British School. He thinks more African students will be there. I'd prefer the International School because I don't want some British public-school type of education for her. And it does the International Baccalaureate, which is spread across more subjects. I like the sound of that. They have a great video on the internet which Isabel and I have looked at. It sounds like a wonderful place.'

Isabel is, however, still resistant to the idea of us going.

'I can't leave you with Uanaingi,' I tell her. Maybe if you were older. But you're 14. You need to be with your parents. And we can't ask Uanaingi to take on the responsibility of driving you to school and afternoon activities, to parties at weekends, and so on. I'm sorry. I know it's hard. But you will meet people there and make new friends. You'll be able to visit interesting places. You'll enjoy it.'

'I won't!' she says. 'I don't want to go! Why are you doing this to me?' She storms off to her room.

I start to sort out old belongings and think about what to take.

'Everything will be provided,' Peter tells me. 'Furniture, linen, kitchen equipment. We only need to take our personal belongings and anything particularly special to us.'

'I want to take our paintings,' I say. We have Namibian art that will make us feel at home.

We decide to let our own house in Windhoek unfurnished, which means we have to pack up everything and store it while we are away. There's a government store for diplomats to use, but we will need help with the packing and transportation. I don't want to contact furniture removal companies yet – Windhoek is too small and people will speculate about what's happening.

'Once my appointment is confirmed, the Foreign Ministry will help us with all that,' Peter says. 'They'll give us names of companies they use, tell us what weight allowance we will have, what can be shipped, etc.'

We need to contact estate agents as well, to find a future tenant, but feel we can't do that yet. It's a strange time of waiting that makes me feel powerless.

I decide to go to take advantage of the delay, and go to the Cape to see Doris and Clive. It's a big step for me, journeying on my own, but I need to see Doris again before I go and I long for the sea.

She picks me up at Cape Town airport, looking relaxed, and gives me a long hug.

'Good to see you,' she says.

'How are you, Doris?' I ask.

'Good, actually, I'm doing well.' It's nine months since she left Windhoek. 'I'm settling in here. It was strange at first, but I love Ceres and I love our house. Can't wait to show it to you.'

We get in her old blue BMW that she had in Windhoek for the past ten years; it still has its Namibian number plates. She drives us through parts of the city I don't know. I'm always disoriented in Cape Town, confused by mountains and sea in different directions, not sure whether I'm facing north, south, east or west, not good at watching the sun for the answer except at the beginning and end of the day. We leave the city and the road leads up through granite mountains, green in parts, with bare grey rock exposed at the top. It's one of the chains of mountains that dominate the landscape around Cape Town. The old car climbs slowly. Doris points out a little spring at the side of the road.

'That's where I come to collect pure water for my babies,' she tells me.

'Babies?'

She laughs: 'Orchids – my new hobby.'

A high mountain pass takes us over the top and into the Ceres valley, and we arrive at their thatched-roof house. Roses flower along the path to the front door. Across the road, a river runs through the trees. It is a softer environment than Windhoek, although Doris tells me she found the summer too hot.

'I loved the winter,' she says. 'It was a real winter, cold and snowy. You can't get through that pass when it's snowed. It reminded me of Germany.' Namibia has desert winters – dry, cold and clear. Temperatures at night drop down to freezing point, but go up to 20 degrees C or more at noon. For three months there's not a cloud in the sky.

There are no demands on me here – no phone, no food to buy, no household tasks or sorting and packing to do, no driving, no children or husband calling on me for anything. Just me and two good friends talking about Namibia, South Africa and the horrors of the Iraq war.

132

Doris has changed from when I saw her last. She's much calmer and doesn't get upset about everything. She and Clive have grown close again.

'I'm still taking medicine,' she tells me, 'and it works well for me.'

'I'm now on four types of pills, in addition to my battery,' I say. 'I find it difficult to think I might have to take them for the rest of my life but they also do their work. What's wrong with us? We are damaged women.'

She shows me an article about women and heart disease.

'Take a look at this,' she says. 'Look at these statistics. What they show is interesting. Most women fear breast cancer, but the figures for that are much lower than those for heart disease. The statistics show that one in three women die of heart disease.'

'So that makes us spot on the statistic,' I respond. 'Two women out of six in our breakfast group with failed hearts. I'm lucky that my heart failure was a type they could do something about.'

Doris invites neighbours they are getting to know, for dinner the next day. I help her chop vegetables and prepare the food but she has always been more organised than me in the kitchen and has little need of help. The other guests include Sheila, a woman in her seventies, who moved to South Africa from Zimbabwe 25 years ago, advised by her doctor to go to a lower altitude after a heart attack. That would have made her 50 at the time, I think, just like me.

'This is my Ceres mother,' Doris says as she introduces Sheila to me. 'She's teaching me how to do tapestry.'

Clive brings us drinks – white wine for Doris and me and a gin and tonic for Sheila. She had been involved in dance and theatre in Zimbabwe and I ask her whether she knew Sandy's family.

She shakes her head. 'I don't think so. But I knew so many people there.'

There's also a middle-aged couple who've recently settled in the Cape – Phil, who is British and his Afrikaner wife, Marie. They have come to the Cape after living in Britain for a long time and they boast about their successful fruit farm.

'Where are you from?' Phil asks me.

'Leeds.'

'The M1 motorway goes to Leeds doesn't it?'

'Yes, I remember when it was finished. Leeds started calling itself "the metropolis of the North". The M1 was the first motorway in England.'

'No,' he says. 'That was another one, near Manchester.' I dispute this and we end up in a silly argument. It makes me feel he's one of those men who knows everything, or thinks he does. When we sit down to eat, Phil talks mostly to Clive, from one end of the table to the other, not listening to or paying attention to the four women in between.

Doris has made pumpkin soup as a starter; it's one of my favourites. I help her clear the bowls when we've finished and bring in lasagne and a large bowl of salad. Clive pours the wine. After a fruit salad dessert, Doris goes into the kitchen to make coffee. The conversation turns to the issue of whites in Africa.

'So Clive,' Phil says, 'do you consider yourself a "white African"?'

'Well, there's the fact that I'm a third generation in this country,' says Clive. 'That gives me the right to use that term. But more than that, I feel that I'm African, and that comes from my travels, especially as a young journalist in the early sixties. I travelled across Africa and the people I met and the way they treated me and received me, made me believe I'm part of this continent.'

'The only problem,' he continues, 'is that I don't really know African culture.'

It's an honest thing to say, since many white Africans claim to know the black Africans so well.

'But what is there really to know?' Phil asks. 'I mean, when Europeans first encountered Africans, they were barbarians. What was there to learn from them?'

I suck in my breath with horror. Do we have to go back to such basics: having to assert that Africans have history, culture and value? I refuse to stoop to that level. Doris comes in to announce that coffee is ready in the sitting room and I stand up, walk to Phil and say:

'That's completely unacceptable, you know,' and I cuff him across the top of his bald head, to admonish him.

He looks up in shock and clearly doesn't understand what I'm objecting to. I walk to the sitting room, not looking at the others, but everyone has gone quiet. Perplexed, Phil follows me. I sit down, still angry but embarrassed now as well. Here I am, about to enter diplomatic life, only to find myself hitting a fellow guest at a dinner party.

'I'm sorry,' I say to Phil, when he comes in and sits down as well. 'I shouldn't have done that. But how can you say there's nothing to learn from African culture? We all have things to learn from each other. People from different times and places have things to offer each other – local knowledge, adaptation to the environment, culture, customs, music, philosophy...'

The grand dame of Zimbabwe agrees with me but we end up having to make the same points I had wanted to rise above.

The next day, Doris, Clive and I drive round the valleys of the Cape, past vineyards and orchards, some of the pear trees still in blossom. We go to the coast, to the De Hoop nature reserve, where we stay in a little white stone fisherman's cottage. That night Clive prepares a fish braai – snoek. It's the most delicious fish I've ever eaten. We eat and drink Cape wine and talk into the night.

In the morning we walk through white sand dunes. A cold wind blows hard from the sea. Doris and I tie on headscarves and I zip my jacket up to the neck to keep out the wind. We find a high point and look out. The sea is rough, with white flurries thrown up by the wind. Huge grey shadows appear beneath the waves: these are the Southern Right whales. They come to the surface and spout water. They leap vertically out of the sea and then dive again, their tails a sharply defined T against the grey. Little ones follow their mothers in the shallower waters. We watch for a long time.

'It makes you know there is a God,' I say to Doris. 'It puts other things into perspective.'

I return to Windhoek refreshed and able to tackle our move.

Peter is formally commissioned by the President in a ceremony at State House. One other ambassador, a woman, is being commissioned at the same time. She will go to Cuba.

'Now Cuba!' Isabel says to me. 'That would be interesting. But Belgium! I don't even know where it is!'

I wear a long royal blue African dress with gold designs down the front. Peter is in his best suit. Isabel, Perivi and Uanaingi come, as well as Uanaingi's daughter Diana and a niece of ours. Isabel wears a little black dress with a high neck buttoned at the side, Chinese style, and her first seriously high-heeled shoes. Perivi is in dark trousers and a tailored African shirt.

It's early morning and already getting hot. We wait in the ante-chamber, where an old stuffed lion from the days before Independence looks at us forlornly, until we are shown in to one of the state rooms. It's long but not very wide, with windows onto a terrace, devoid of furniture that has been removed to make room for everyone, except for one table and chair. It's the same room in which we had the reception to send off the South African Administrator General 13 years ago.

The protocol people have briefed Peter on the proceedings but I'm still not sure what to expect. They are there in numbers, quietly telling us what we should be doing, where to stand and where to go. I must stand beside Peter, and the children behind us. As he is called, I must take a step back.

When everyone is in place, President Sam Nujoma, his wife, and the Foreign Minister and his wife, come in from a side room. The President calls Peter up and gives him the letters of credence, on embossed state letterheads, stating his appointment. Peter will hand these over to the Heads of State of the countries to which he is now posted. Peter bows and shakes hands with the President and Foreign Minister. He moves to the podium, reads the official oath of office and signs the book. He makes a few remarks, pledging to serve Namibia to the best of his ability in his new role. Then he goes round the room, beaming, shaking hands with people, and comes to stand with us.

The heat has got to Isabel and she looks as if she is going to faint. We ask for a chair so she can sit down. Someone brings one, and a glass of water.

The next ambassador goes through the same procedures. She's dressed in a cream tailored African suit with brown geometric patterns, sleeves puffed at the shoulder, an ankle-length straight skirt, a matching scarf tied like a little pill-box hat on the top of her head. Peter joins her and they stand with the President and Foreign Minister for official photos at the back of the room, in front of a vast painting of Epupa Falls, on the Kunene River, Namibia's northern border with Angola. Afterwards the President goes round the room, shaking hands with everyone. As he approaches us, Perivi hisses at Isabel:

'Get up. Stand up for the President!'

He graciously assures her that she may remain seated.

We move onto the terrace for light refreshments – delicate sandwiches and small sausage rolls, soft drinks and champagne. The fresh air and food revive Isabel. Members of the press outside ask Peter for comments and take more photos. A press statement is released. It is official. We are going. Soon.

Sitting on Deedee's balcony, soaking in my friends – Deedee, Jane and Sandy. How many more times will we sit together like this?

The table is covered with empty cups. Deedee puts them on a tray and takes them into the house. She comes back with a bottle of cold white wine and glasses. She opens the wine and starts to pour it, handing a glass to each of us.

'I need ice,' says Sandy.

'You know where it is. Can you bring some out?' Deedee asks her. Sandy gets up to do so.

Jane is looking tired. 'What's going on?' we ask her.

'I have to tell you, I'm in shock,' she says. 'I've just heard about the loss of a niece who died from malaria. She was lovely – one of my real favourites. And she's gone. Just like that. It was quick and it was completely unexpected.'

'Oh, Jane, we're so sorry,' Deedee speaks and we echo her words.

Jane's eyes fill with tears.

'I'm just so used to hearing about deaths from AIDS these days that I forget there are other things that can take one too,' she says.

Jane has spearheaded the leadership of HIV-positive people, hiring them to lead and plan HIV/AIDS campaigns. Deedee is helping to develop strategic plans for dealing with HIV/AIDS. Sandy workshops poems and songs with young people as part of a school AIDS awareness campaign. We all know people who are positive. We know people who have died from this disease. It reaches into all our lives.

I tell them about my trip to the Cape and the dinner at Doris and Clive's. I tell Sandy about Sheila, the woman from Zimbabwe.

'I wondered if she knew your family, but she said she didn't. Maybe you knew of her? She told me that her husband was responsible for building the Kariba Dam.'

'Along with x thousand others,' Sandy points out.

I tell them what their other guest said and that I hit him on the head.

'Well done!' says Jane and we burst out laughing.

We were planning an overnight stay at a lodge together, as our farewell, but I tell them I can't make it. I've broken our arrangement out of loyalty to Peter. Anyone else, any other social arrangement would have been second to this planned time together with my friends, but there is to be a staff farewell at the University for Peter that night and it wouldn't seem right if I missed it.

There is a sequence of farewell dinners, including a formal one given by the University, to which government ministers and officials, diplomats, businessmen and women and other educationalists are invited. We have a family table for Perivi, Isabel, Uanaingi and Kavesorere, Peter's sisters, and Alexia. Peter and I have to sit at a long high table, looking out at the room, confined to speak only to those each side of us, aware that we are on display while we eat. There are old friends with us at the table, including Sandra and Mosé, the Prime Minister Theo-Ben Gurirab and his wife Joan. There's a succession of messages from the Prime Minister, the incoming Vice Chancellor and the Rector of the Polytechnic, all of them saying wonderful things about Peter and his work at the University.

There is also a party given by the American Ambassador, mooted at a previous reception where Peter and the ambassador had challenged each other to a karaoke session. The planning for it goes ahead.

'The karaoke part is really not necessary,' I tell the ambassador's wife. I'm very worried about it but the men are committed, even though neither of them has ever done this before. We find a local musician who knows how to set it up, and who has the words for various popular songs. He has done karaoke sessions before and knows how to draw people in and propose different songs. This makes me feel a little less nervous.

The night arrives, and the karaoke session takes in ambassadors and government ministers alike. Michael dons a shoulder-length blond wig, and starts to sing. A top legal adviser to the government fights him for the microphone. Peter and I sing 'My Way'. Deedee, Sandy and Jane prove to be good back-up dancers. I get caught up in it and try to encourage Jane and Helao to join us in singing 'Ebony and Ivory'.

'I don't think so,' she says.

'A bit tacky?' I ask her.

'Yes.'

Perivi and Isabel are with us and they cannot believe what they see. All the uncles who tell them not to stay out late or do crazy things are letting their hair down.

'I have enough information tonight to topple the Government,' jokes Perivi.

And I find that I can dance. My pacemaker is sensitive to movement, and speeds up when I am moving on the dance-floor, giving me the extra oxygen I need.

Before we leave, I visit Hugo and give him my copy of Fauré's Requiem that I listened to so much a year ago.

'It takes you into the sorrow and then through it.' I tell him, and also give him a copy of the prayer I read at Brigitte's memorial, the one that Isobel liked so much.

I think long and hard about something to give Sandy, Deedee and Jane. Nothing seems appropriate and in the end I decide on pieces of my favourite jewellery – a string of blue Indonesian pearls that I tell Deedee she must share with Tricia; a necklace of chunks of amber for Sandy that Peter had given me a few years before, that I love; and a carved bone necklace for Jane that I bought in the Mall near my bookshop, and that reminds me of that part of my life.

'I read that jewellery retains something of the owner's spirit,' I tell them. 'This way, some of my spirit will remain here with you.'

At Sandy's we have the final farewell, with our husbands, sitting on the deck at a long wooden table in the light of a huge full moon, the hills of Windhoek outlined against the sky. It's November, and it's warm outside at night. There's a Jacuzzi below the deck and Sandy, Jane, Deedee and I get in, the water bubbling, our glasses of champagne bubbling, talking and laughing on our last evening together, ignoring the fact that everything we say is rising to the ears of the men seated above. There is so much that I want to say, so many words that clog my throat.

'I'm going to miss you all so much. This has been the best group of friends I've ever had. I've never known such friendship and I am enriched by it.

'But I know I will make other friends over there,' I say. 'I've had your love and now I know how to share it.'

Wrenching ourselves out of Windhoek is acutely painful. We spend the last two nights in a hotel but the process of sorting things out doesn't seem to stop until we head off for the airport. We leave in a convoy of vehicles – Peter and I, Perivi and Isabel, with a collection of large suitcases to check in and nine pieces of hand luggage between us. Family and friends follow and Peter's closest colleagues from his office. We're late and we phone ahead to the airport to ask them to keep the checking-in desk open for us. Perivi is excited. Peter is stressed. I weep as we drive to the airport. I feel as if I'm being ripped out of the land. Isabel weeps on the plane until she becomes transfixed by the display of clouds: grey, fluffy and white, banking as the heat builds up in the afternoon, the edges lit by yellow shafts of sunshine, and small pockets of rain – all too rare a sight in Namibia.

PART 3

A whole new world

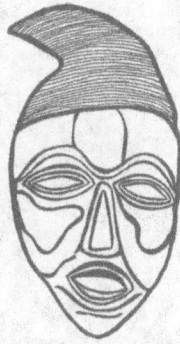

The house sits in the midst of greenery: a mock-Georgian rectangle of white stone with a flat roof and vast lawn, complete with flagpole in the middle. A weeping willow drapes round one corner of the house. Rhododendron bushes mass at the side of the driveway and along the edge of the lawn; silver birches and enormous fir trees border the back of the garden. Automatic wrought-iron gates bearing the coat of arms of Namibia open onto a circular drive that goes round the back of the house and out through similar gates on the other side of the garden.

I have seen photos of the house before but nothing prepares me for the size of it. We're driven up to the front door. The chauffeur stops the ambassadorial black Mercedes, gets out and unlocks the door of the house. He opens the car doors for Peter and me to get out, and shows us into the house. Perivi and Isabel arrive behind us in one of the other embassy cars. Our luggage is in a third.

We enter the house. A large diamond-shaped chandelier hangs low in the centre of a high-ceilinged entrance hall. To the left stands a Namibian flag, two metres tall. To the right, a circular staircase with ornate metal railing sweeps up to the first floor. Three adjoining reception rooms open up in front of us, with French windows that lead onto the lawn. There's a breakfast room, a large kitchen, a study at the bottom of the stairs with a large wooden desk, a cloakroom and guest toilet to the right of the front door.

I look at Peter and raise my eyebrows. He smiles but says nothing; he has visited the residence before.

'Okay,' says Perivi quietly, drawing out the word.

While the drivers bring in our luggage, we go into the main sitting room. Two beige leather sofas with elegant wooden arms are placed round a low rectangular coffee table. Two matching chairs are at one end; two others with beige and pink tapestry upholstery are at the other. In the adjoining dining room stands a large table with ten chairs, a dark polished cabinet and heavy matching sideboard.

All the walls are painted white; the curtains are a pale pink. Framed photos of Namibian landscapes hang high on the walls but are lost in the sheer size of everything.

A short Filipino woman with shoulder-length black hair comes towards us. She wears black trousers and a thigh-length, mustard-coloured top. The chauffeur introduces us.

'This is the housekeeper, Concepcion. She's been with the embassy since it was opened 13 years ago. She's looked after all the ambassadors.'

'Good morning Ambassador, good morning Madame,' she says and gives us a broad smile.

Concepcion leads us up the stairs – Peter and me, Perivi, Isabel, two drivers, two other embassy staff; the whole group going round to explore each room. She opens doors in the corridor to show us the large linen cupboards where towels and sheets are stored. There's a bathroom at one end of the corridor and a toilet at the other end. Two bedrooms are at the back of the house, one with its own bathroom, the other with another room opening from it, and from that, a toilet and narrow stairs that lead down to a door next to the kitchen; it was built to be used by a maid. The front of the house has three double bedrooms. In the middle, at the top of the stairs, is the master bedroom, a large room with French windows that open onto a very narrow balcony, a wall of built-in cupboards, an en-suite shower and separate en-suite bathroom. Again, everything is painted white. There's basic furniture in all the rooms but the absence of personal belongings makes the house seem very bare; the absence of colour makes it feel cold.

We go downstairs again and into the kitchen. Concepcion opens the cupboards. They are almost empty, except for a few plates that don't match, cracked mugs, three saucepans, and a collection of everyday knives, forks and spoons. The previous ambassador left two months before our arrival and there is no food at all, not even salt, pepper or sugar. The Counsellor at the embassy had warned us of this, and we stopped on our way from the airport to pick up essential supplies: coffee, tea, bread, ham, cheese and fruit.

'Which bedroom do you want, Isabel? I ask. 'You're spoilt for choice.'

'The two rooms at the back with the stairs,' she says. We go up to have another look. A huge black, shining wardrobe, with a full-length mirror in the middle, covers one wall of the bedroom.

'Well, you'll have plenty of space for your clothes,' I say to her. 'And you can use one room as your bedroom and the other as a study,' I add. 'You have private stairs for going to the kitchen and having midnight feasts without us knowing.'

144

'Or going out late and coming back without you knowing,' she replies, with a little smile.

Perivi chooses one of the front bedrooms, with a white dressing table and mirror, and white headboard and bedside tables. He claims his luggage and starts to unpack. Peter and I move into the master bedroom. It has the rest of the black shining bedroom set: a headboard with bedside cupboards, matching dressing table, and a television on a black table. The carpet is pale green. The combined effect, against the white walls, is cold and hard. The walls of the bathroom that leads off it are covered with minute pale blue tiles; the shower room with similar pink tiles. All the beds have been made up by Concepcion. The top of the duvet cover on ours is white satin, but it has been darned.

I choose one of the other bedrooms that overlook the garden as my future study, but have nothing to put in it yet. We brought clothes and family files, and CDs for Perivi and Isabel in our luggage on the plane. Isabel also packed her purple duvet cover and pillowcases. Other personal belongings are still on their way to us by sea: a few mementos from Isabel's room at home, my favourite artwork, a variety of reference books for Peter and me, and all the family photos that I want to sort out while I'm here. I also packed our old records from the 1970s and 1980s; I think I can get them copied onto CDs in Europe, so we can listen to them once again.

Apart from the few pieces we saw in the kitchen, the crockery and cutlery have been locked away for safety by the previous ambassador. It takes three days for the embassy staff to find the keys, so during that time we lead a mixture of high life and low, carrying early morning tea upstairs in mugs that have no handles, on a silver tray that was left in the dining room cabinet.

We are not shown how things work – where the fuse box is, how to light the boiler, or where to find spare light bulbs. These and other secrets of the house are kept by Concepcion, who has worked there since it was bought by our embassy ten years ago. Concepcion speaks a little English and a little French but she is partly deaf, and it's difficult to communicate with her. She moves quietly round the house as she cleans each day. She takes dirty clothes down to the basement and washes and irons them there. I go down to see. There's a large room with an ironing board, a sofa and two chairs in it, and a small washing room with washing lines strung across it that have clothes drying on them. The atmosphere is damp.

'Why don't we hang the clothes out in the fresh air?' I ask Concepcion. I'm used to clothes drying very quickly in Namibia.

'Yes Madame,' she says but doesn't do it.

I try to put my stamp on the house by rearranging some of the furniture in the sitting room.

'I'd like the sofas this way, Concepcion,' I say to her.

'Yes Madame,' she replies but moves them back to where they were before.

'Please don't put the pot plants in the hearth,' I ask her. 'The cold draft coming down the chimney isn't good for them.'

'Yes Madame,' she says but nothing changes.

'It's clear Concepcion has her own way of doing things,' I say to Peter.

'Well, she's worked for two ambassadors here before us,' he replies.

'So she knows she will be here when we've gone,' I say. He smiles.

Concepcion stays with her son and his family in Mechelen, outside Brussels. She travels to work very early in the morning by train and tram. We never hear or see her arrive. When I go downstairs at seven in the morning to make a cup of tea, the light is already on in the basement and she is there. If I go down at six to get a glass of cold water from the fridge, she is also there.

'Perhaps she's really living in the basement,' I say to Peter.

'It's possible,' he replies, but there is no evidence of it.

I ask Concepcion to take me into the flat behind the garage. I don't know where the key is but she finds it and we go over. There are two large doors side by side in the corner of an L-shaped building that comprises the garage and flat. One door leads to a tiny two-roomed flat with its own bathroom. It smells damp, the carpets are old and stained and the taps in the bathroom don't run. The second door leads into a larger flat with kitchen, bedroom, bathroom and a large reception room that overlooks the garden. Again, it smells damp. There are marks on the walls where water has run down from the ceiling and the plaster has bubbles in it from water damage. We check the basement. Old chairs and broken coffee tables are stored down there but the floor is flooded.

The house itself also has problems. There are places where the roof leaks and the washing room in the basement floods after a bad storm one weekend. The shower in our pink en-suite bathroom doesn't work properly and no water comes when we turn on the taps in our bathroom. We use one of the other bathrooms but calcium in the water has stained the basins and baths with brown marks over the years.

'Can't you scrub them away?' I ask Concepcion.

'I tried, Madame,' she tells me, 'but they won't go.' We buy strong cleaning products and Concepcion tries to clean the baths that way, but it makes no difference. Peter and I compile a list of things that need repairing and he reports back to our Ministry for Foreign Affairs and asks for funds.

Isabel stays at home with us for a week as we adjust to our new environment. After that, she is due to start at the International School. It's late in the autumn term and there's only four weeks before the Christmas break, but I think that will be good for her. She can have Christmas to look forward to as she gets used to the place.

I arrange to visit the school with her before she starts. Peter's chauffeur, Mamadou, collects us from the residence in the black Mercedes. He drives us down avenues lined with tall trees, past decorative art nouveau houses from the early twentieth century, until we come to the school itself – a collection of modern buildings around an old square house, set in a park with tall trees. We go to the central administrative office and report there. They direct us across the park to the secondary school, to meet one of the teachers responsible for that section.

It's the middle of the morning and children of all ages are walking between buildings or playing on the basketball courts, chattering noisily. We hear a little French but the predominant language is English; the predominant accent is American. The children look as if they come from countries in Europe, the Americas and Asia; there are very few black faces.

We go into an office to meet the teacher responsible for Isabel's grade, an American in his mid-thirties. He asks Isabel about herself and gives her a timetable.

'You're in Grade 9,' he tells her. 'Come to this building on Monday morning and find yourself a locker. You get a padlock from the office. The timetable tells you where each lesson is. The other students will help you find where you need to go.'

'I don't want to be in Grade 9,' she tells me as we leave the building. She has just finished Grade 9 in Windhoek and was expecting to go into Grade 10 as a late starter.

'The numbering system here is different,' I try to reassure her. 'It's not the same as Grade 9 in Windhoek. It will be Grade 10 work.' But I'm already wondering if this is the right place for her.

A school bus picks Isabel up from outside the gates to the residence at 7.30 the following Monday and brings her back at 5.00, at the end of the school day.

'How did it go?' I ask her. 'The first day is always the worst, you know.'

'It wasn't too bad. I didn't know where to go or what to do, though.'

After the second day, I ask her again how it went.

'It was dreadful!'

The third day is worse. She comes home looking pale.

'I don't know anyone,' she says. 'I didn't have anyone to sit with at lunchtime. I just hung around the lockers.'

The fourth day the nurse phones me from school to tell me Isabel isn't feeling well.

'She's got a headache and stomach ache,' says the nurse. 'I think you'd better fetch her.' I phone Peter at the embassy and he sends Mamadou to bring her home. She returns looking miserable and goes to her room to lie down. The next day, she refuses to get up.

I phone the school and speak to the teacher we met. 'I'm not sure how to handle this,' I tell him.

'She's arrived at a difficult time, three-quarters of the way through the term, when friendships have already been formed,' he responds. 'It'll take time but she'll settle in.'

'I hate it!' she tells me. 'I feel completely left out.'

'I know it must be hard,' I say. 'But I'm sure you'll be alright in the end. You can stay at home another day. Then you must go back and try again.'

She returns to school but each day she comes home looking drawn. She has less and less to say to us. She is given an essay and a poem to write for an English assignment, and she writes about slavery, and about being forcibly taken across the seas, away from her home. She shows them to me before she hands them in. I'm shocked at the depth of her anguish.

I approach Sophia, the Counsellor at our embassy; she has a daughter Isabel's age who is at the British School.

'Do you think there'd be space for Isabel there?' I ask her. She enquires and gives me the name and number of the person to talk to.

'If she comes straight away, it should be possible,' they tell me. There's two weeks of term left. 'We don't accept people in January because they will have missed too much. But if she comes now, we can give her work to catch up on over the holiday.'

Isabel's teacher at the International School thinks she will fit in there if she stays, and will still be homesick for Namibia if she goes to the British School.

'Maybe,' I say to him. 'But she feels we've dragged her here against her will. This is the one thing she can decide for herself.'

I take Isabel to the British School. It's another series of modern buildings, located in the grounds of the former palace of the Belgian King Leopold II, notorious for the brutality of his rule of the Congo in the late nineteenth and early twentieth centuries.

The atmosphere at the school is friendly. The accents are regional British ones, and Isabel smiles at me with recognition as she hears them. The teachers we meet explain the system there, which is almost the same as the Namibian one that Isabel has come out of. They are informal and helpful. It's quite unlike what I had feared when we were trying to choose which school to apply to. I had thought the British School might be conservative, disciplinarian and snobby, as private British schools were when I was growing up, but it isn't like that at all.

Isabel starts at the British School two weeks after starting at the International School. There's also a school bus, which goes from the end of our road. She's in the same year, but not the same class as Sophia's daughter Shali, who introduces Isabel to other African girls at the school who are her age. They take Isabel under their wing. They meet up with other teenagers, mostly from African embassies, show her the shops in town, and how to use the tram that passes near our house.

Perivi also finds a friend, Jerome, the son of one of our other embassy officials. Jerome is in the middle of a law degree in South Africa but is in Brussels for a year. He takes Perivi round the clubs and introduces him to other young people he knows. One night we are woken by a phone call from Perivi at one in the morning.

'Can you come and get me?' he asks. 'I got off the tram at the wrong place and that was the last tram,'

We groan and ask 'Where are you?'

'I don't know,' he replies. Peter and I get dressed, get out the Mercedes and trawl slowly down the tram route until we find our son, sitting alone in a shelter under the trees.

The residence lies on the edge of the Forét de Soignes, the largest surviving beech forest in Europe. Napoleon marched here 190 years ago on his way to the Battle of Waterloo. The battle ground itself is now a museum site. The small adjacent town of Waterloo is 20 minutes drive from where we live.

Trams rattle through the forest. Isabel's school is in one direction, the centre of town in the other. It's Isabel who takes us on our first tram journey there. We change from tram to the underground metro system at a stop named Montgomery after British Field Marshal Montgomery, who led Allied forces in the liberation of Belgian cities. We get off at the central station. Muslim women wearing headscarves or the fuller hijab that covers hair, head, and shoulders, walk by. Eastern European women with bright rose-patterned scarves sit by the station entrance, cups in hand, sometimes a baby on their knees, asking for money.

We walk down to the 'old town', an area of narrow cobbled streets and alleyways, with lace shops, chocolateries, and restaurants. We turn into Grand Place, the ancient heart of Brussels, a cobbled square surrounded by tall, narrow, seventeenth-century buildings with elaborate gables decorated in gold, and a beautiful, ornate white town hall with spire. We choose one of the restaurants on the square. I order beef stew with mash potatoes and carrots while Peter, Perivi and Isabel have steak and Belgian fries. At the table next to us, a man is tackling a huge bowl of mussels, forking them out of their shells and into his mouth.

On another day, Mamadou drives us round more of the city, past the modern blocks of the headquarters of the European Commission and other EU offices. The new EU Parliament buildings have huge glass walls.

'To aid transparency,' we are told by a Member of the European Parliament, when we visit.

The streets and the population begin to change behind the EU buildings. The mostly white faces of EU officials give way to brown and black. There are rows of small terrace houses and corner shops. A little further on, the shops increase in number. The vegetables laid out in racks include yams, sweet potatoes and okra. Plantain hangs in clumps from hooks – green or darkened yellow. Other shops sell cloth from West Africa and cafés list African specialities on their windows. A huge mural on one wall claims that this is Matonge, home to people from many different nationalities and languages, predominantly African. It's named after the marketplace and commercial district of the same name in Kinshasa, capital of the Congo.

'Can I get a haircut here?' Peter asks and Mamadou arranges to bring him later.

'And me?' asks Isabel. Mamadou takes Isabel and me back to Matonge another day to explore. Down the arcades are barbers and hairdressers with photos of elaborate braided hairstyles or wigs in the window. The models and the hairdressers are black.

'Can I get my hair braided?' Isabel asks me.

'Sure,' I reply. She's braided her hair before but not for over a year.

We pick a tiny hairdressing salon and find that the woman in charge is from the Cameroon, and speaks English as well as French. Isabel is relieved. I help her explain what she wants to the hairdresser – very fine long braids – and sit with her until the braiding starts. Then I walk round the nearby shops, have a coffee, and go back to see how Isabel is doing. It's a long process and she isn't ready. I go out again and walk a bit further, round the corner from the Matonge mural, and on to the Boulevard de Waterloo. It's immediately different, an exclusive shopping area of designer clothes stores and women in expensive looking suits.

I go back again to see how Isabel is doing. Five hours after her appointment started, her hairstyle is finished. The thin braids pull her hair back from her face and hang down at the sides. A lighter brown strand has been woven in with the black and gives depth to the colour.

'You look beautiful,' I tell her and she gives me a broad smile. I phone Mamadou and get him to pick us up.

The official palace of the ruling monarch lies beyond the expensive shopping district, with a formally laid out park right in front that used to be part of the palace grounds, but is now open to the public. This palace is where Peter will present his letters of credence from President Nujoma to King Albert II. Only after that will he be able to take up his duties.

On the appointed day, two black Mercedes and three police motorbike outriders arrive at the residence and stop outside the front door. Mamadou opens it and shows in the King's Marshall. He wears a grey-blue dress uniform with gold braids strung across his chest.

'I have been sent by the King to collect Professor Peter Katjavivi,' the Marshall announces formally, standing by the Namibian flag in the entrance hall. Peter is ready, dressed in tails and a white bowtie hired from a gentleman's tailor that serves the diplomatic community.

'You look magnificent! Tall and elegant.' I told him when he put it on earlier, and he smiled proudly.

Now he steps forward to join the Marshall. Sophia and two other diplomats from our embassy go with them. The car that Peter travels in flies the Namibian flag and it flutters in the wind as they sweep down the drive. The traffic stops as they drive through the city and when they get near to the palace, an escort of horsemen and horsewomen replace the outriders and lead them in. Afterwards they all, including the Marshall, come back to the residence for champagne and canapés. We take photos of Peter and the Marshall, and then the four of us in front of the flag in the entrance hall. Perivi is dressed in a plum-coloured African shirt and dark trousers. I wear a smart new woolen jacket with square blocks of bright colours on a black background and an ankle-length black skirt, both of which I bought for the occasion, even though I did not accompany Peter. Isabel, unfortunately, is at school.

'So what happened at the palace?' I ask Peter later.

'We were led into the anteroom and from there into another room where the King was,' he says. 'I was formally introduced and I stepped towards him, holding my letter of credentials, and presented myself. The King accepted the letter and we took a photo. Then he indicated that I should sit with him.'

'What did you talk about?'

'He asked me how things are in Namibia since Independence, and I talked in general for a while,' Peter replies. 'But I wanted to convey a specific message from President Nujoma to him, as well.'

'What was that?'

'President Nujoma asked me to send his greetings to the King and through him to the people of Belgium,' Peter says. 'He asked me to recall the support of individuals and organizations in Belgium for the liberation struggle in Namibia, and he asked me to convey an invitation to the King to come and visit Namibia.'

'And was the King interested?' I ask.

'Well, I think so,' Peter says. 'It's the first step, of course, but we have to invite him more formally now and see what we can arrange.'

Christmas approaches but I don't want to think about last Christmas, about Isobel's heart attack forever staining the day for Hugo and their children. So I seek comfort in my family in England. Peter, Perivi, Isabel and I travel to Bristol, in the southwest of England, to stay with my elder sister, Sarah, her husband Dennis, and their children, who are in their early twenties.

Sarah is an educationalist in multicultural Britain, heading a programme to empower inner-city Bristol schools and children disadvantaged because of their race and class. Dennis is a former hospital administrator, committed to serving the community, now working in the local high court since Sarah's job brought them to Bristol. Their three children are very creative. Rachel is a textile artist, Martin an animator, and Alison a classical double bass player who does concerts with different orchestras and teaches double bass as well. For ten years, Sarah and Dennis also fostered two brothers with a white mother and black fathers, who had been violently abused when they were young.

It is seven years since we celebrated Christmas in Europe. The short days and dark wet weather are such a contrast to the heat in Namibia. The winter atmosphere fits in with the traditional images of snow, fir trees and reindeer that still grace Christmas cards in the shops in Windhoek. The Christmas decorations in Brussels are elegant – little white lights on Christmas trees outside each shop. The lights in Britain are more garish. The consumerism in both countries is so much greater than in Namibia, the shopping crowds pervasive. Presents are not a big part of Christmas in Namibia. It's usually a time to spend with family, in the village or on the farm.

'I remember the smell of oranges at Christmas,' Peter tells Perivi and Isabel. 'That's what I was given as a child. That was our treat.'

At Sarah's we have a traditional English Christmas turkey but also vegetarian dishes as well: her children do not eat meat. We go for a walk the next day and look at the Bristol suspension bridge, made of iron, an engineering feat of the nineteenth century, built by Isambard Kingdom Brunel in Britain's industrial heyday.

For New Year's Eve, Perivi travels by coach to visit Namibian friends in London. Peter, Isabel and I go to stay with my parents in their house near Oxford, where they retired soon after we went to live in Namibia, and we celebrate quietly with them there.

My mother Ruth is slim and fit through gardening almost every day, even in the winter; she bends almost double to pull out the weeds. At 83, she is still naturally dark-haired.

'I have more grey hair than you do, you know' I tell her as we sit in the kitchen, warmed by the Aga cooker, drinking coffee in the morning.

'But your hair looks pretty, Jane,' she says.

'Thanks, but it's not natural. It's got highlights and lowlights to look like this. You're lucky,' I tell her.

A natural linguist and lover of literature, Ruth quotes from the classics whenever a conversation or phrase taps into her literary knowledge, far greater than mine even though I studied Literature at university. When she was unable to go to university because of the War, she applied for a job in the civil service, and worked there until 1947, the year she and my father were married. She lost her job then because the civil service wouldn't employ married women in those days, and she dedicated her life to family, looking after us and both my grandmothers in the last ten years of their lives. She also assisted various charities.

My father John is a loving, loyal man who took over the family business from his father after fighting in the Far East during the War. He too, loves literature but he focussed on the business, as a wholesale paper merchant, buying paper from the mills and selling it on to printers and local schools. When the printers started to buy directly from the mills in the 1960s, the middlemen like my father lost customers, but he kept the business going through difficult times, and made sure we had the education we needed to get to university.

After my grandmother died aged 101, a year after Isabel was born, my parents moved to the farmhouse where my mother's parents had lived, and where we used to go for holidays when we were children. They built on an extension to give the house more bedrooms, and brought their furniture down from Leeds. The result was a merging of the two houses of my childhood.

At the bottom of the drive are the remains of an old railway line. My mother travelled to school on that line in the 1930s and we used to watch the steam trains that ran there once a day in the 1950s; it was closed down a decade later. On the other side of the railway line is a small wood of willow trees planted by my grandfather, who wanted to sell them to make cricket bats. Near the drive are three large fir trees that have grown from Christmas trees we planted when we were children.

'It's beautifully calm here,' I tell Ruth as we look out over the garden on New Year's Day. 'It's such a lovely place.'

'Thank you, my dear,' she says, and asks 'Do you do any gardening in Brussels?'

'No, none,' I tell her. 'I like to look at gardens and sit in them and I keep thinking I'll do some gardening myself, but I've never really done so.'

'Perhaps it's something you could enjoy now that you're not working,' she says.

'Perhaps.'

She switches tack: 'What do you want this year to bring, Jane?' she asks me. 'Got any resolutions?'

'Not really,' I reply. 'I just want 2004 to be a better year than the last.'

'Travel hopefully,' she advises me.

We return to Brussels and Perivi prepares to leave to pursue his own studies in Syracuse, in up-state New York. He is to stay with friends who teach at the same college. I book him a ticket from the Charles de Gaulle airport in Paris, directly to New York, and Mamadou drives us there to see Perivi off. We arrange to stay in a hotel at the airport the night before, as his flight leaves very early in the morning.

The day before Perivi is due to travel, a number of flights to the USA are cancelled. American security services are now checking the names of all those booked on flights to US cities, and they don't like the name of one of the passengers due to travel that day; they think it might be someone on their lists of suspected terrorist sympathisers. We proceed anxiously to the airport, not sure whether Perivi's flight will also be cancelled, check into the hotel and have dinner together. We get up at five in the morning and go into the airport, looking around for the flight announcements. Fortunately, the flight is listed; there are no cancellations and no problems with Perivi's check-in.

We sit down for a coffee, feeling tired and not wanting to say goodbye.

'Perivi, I want you to be serious about your studies,' Peter tells him. 'There are lots of people your age who would love the chance to go to America to study. Take this opportunity and use it to your advantage.'

'I'm excited,' says Perivi. 'This is the next stage of my journey. I'm looking forward to it.'

'I want to tell you so much, to wish you well, and give you advice, and tell you what to do and what to watch out for,' I say. 'But I think you know everything I would say.'

'I'm going to miss you,' Isabel tells him.

We stand up to walk with Perivi towards the security gate he must pass through, and we hug him farewell. Mamadou, not much taller than Perivi, slightly stocky, with a neat moustache, puts his right hand over his heart and addresses Perivi directly.

'Remember why you are there and you will be alright,' he says, 'Insha'Allah.'

We wave Perivi through the security check.

'Let's hope he's alright,' I say to Peter when Perivi has disappeared from view. I pause. 'You know, we're here in Paris, now. Let's show Isabel a bit of Paris.'

'Alright,' he says, and Mamadou takes us on an impromptu tour, stopping for us to get out at the Eiffel Tower and take photos. We have lunch at a small restaurant nearby and enjoy steak, chips and salad.

'I used to live in Paris,' Mamadou tells us. 'My uncle was a Senegalese diplomat there in the 1960s.' He proceeds to tell us about his uncle's role in Senegalese politics and the contribution of troops from Senegal and other Francophone West African countries to France's army during the Second World War.

We return to Brussels that evening, amazed that we can do a trip like this within 24 hours. A few days later, we read in the newspaper that the passenger whose name the Americans had been worried about was an elderly Chinese woman, not an actual security threat.

I phone Windhoek a few days later, on the anniversary of Isobel's death, the day in early January when Hugo and the children were to bring her back to Windhoek, when what was supposed to be a journey of homecoming turned into a journey to her grave. This is a day when my friends and I would have come together to remember Isobel and talk about her, to hold her family in our thoughts.

I try to get hold of Deedee, Jane or Sandy but can find no one – they must still be away on their summer holidays. Sandy's voice comes on her answer-phone and it so unnerves me that my tears begin to flow. How near and yet how far my friends are! I long for them.

The next day, a few shafts of weak sunlight filter through the trees.

'Let's go for a walk,' suggests Peter.

The sun disappears as soon as we get outside and a cold wind picks up. We walk towards a small square near the residence, with a church, a few shops and a market on Wednesdays. A path leads to it down an alleyway between large gardens. We follow the path and emerge on the edge of a ploughed field, with stalks scattered on the soil.

'Let me see what crop was in the field,' I say, thinking I can show off my limited knowledge of cereal farming, gleaned from my grandfather. I pick up some of the stalks, but I can't identify them. Peter bends down and picks up a discarded husk.

'They're mealies,' he says, surprised. It's the staple diet for southern Africa.

'That makes me feel at home,' Peter says.

I suddenly feel connected. I think about Isobel and know that she would have enjoyed Brussels. She would have been busy visiting the art galleries, the coffee shops and chocolate shops, the museums and exhibitions. I can take her with me in my heart and begin to enjoy it as well.

When we return to the house, I check for emails on Peter's computer in his study, and find one from Deedee. She tells me they are going to gather this weekend at the farm where Isobel is buried, in remembrance of her. I can see them, Deedee and Sandy, standing on top of the hill by Isobel's grave, the evening sun sending low shards of light across the landscape, between the rain clouds, for it is raining now in Namibia. They are talking quietly to and about Isobel. I touch her grave through their fingers, in respect and love. Then I see them weeping. I weep with them. There is nothing else to do but weep, then get up and carry on.

We have heard from friends and family that it's raining heavily in Namibia, an outpouring of water on a scale unseen for 100 years. It is impossible to tell someone who has not lived in a dry land what rain feels like after eight or nine months of clear skies. That mad feeling when people rush out of their houses and cars and seek the soaking. When women hoist their skirts and wade into the flood rushing down a dry riverbed, hypnotised by the water, ignorant of the fact that they might be taken up and swept away forever. If it is raining in Namibia, then it should be a good year.

In Brussels, the rain slants across the window in thick sheets, pouring into the bright green sponge of the lawn below. The trees push up, outlined against a surreal white sky; their trunks sway and lean over as the wind bears down upon them. Twigs fly past and add to those already scattered over the drive. The wind circles the house.

'It's too cold for me,' I tell Peter. 'I may have grown up in winters like this but I'm no longer adapted to them.'

'It's too cold and wet for Isabel to take the bus to school,' says Peter and arranges for Pascal, the second embassy driver, to take her and bring her home.

At 8.00 in the morning, while I am still in my dressing gown, having breakfast, Pascal arrives. He wears a cap and scarf but takes his cap off when he sees me.

'*Bonjour* Madame,' he says. '*Bonjour* Isabel.' They climb into the car, turn to the left out of our gate, and join the Avenue de Tervuren that will take them to Isabel's school.

At 8.30, Mamadou arrives to collect Peter.

'Good morning, Madame. Good morning Excellency,' he says. He opens the car door for Peter, who gets in the back, on the opposite side. They turn to the right out of our gate and head for the embassy, which also lies on the Avenue de Tervuren, but further towards town; it's a ten-minute drive.

The embassy is a self-contained, square, modern two-storey building in an area where other embassies are also located. The embassy of the People's Republic of China is opposite ours. Demonstrators frequently stand in the tree-lined centre of the Avenue, with signs directed at the Chinese Embassy, protesting human rights abuses.

Peter takes to diplomatic life very easily. He assesses his new tasks and his new colleagues. He meets other ambassadors, Members of the European Parliament, businessmen and women, and talks to everyone, everywhere, about Namibia.

It takes time for me to find my way. Thrown into a new environment, I don't have networks of friends or family or work. But after all the planning and packing before our departure from Windhoek, I'm glad I don't have much to do. I start to read again. In the afternoons I watch daytime TV for the first time in my life – there are so many channels available in Brussels. I settle into a comfy chair in our bedroom, with my feet up, and choose gentle English murder mysteries and home improvement or garden shows. I doze in the chair, or lie down on the bed and sleep until 4 p.m. From 4.30 I sit at the study window, watching and waiting for Peter and Isabel to return.

When our goods arrive from Namibia, I unpack. I sort books, family photos and files, put Peter's into his study and mine into my study upstairs. I take the existing photos off the walls and hang our artwork in the reception rooms and on the landing. Most of it is by Namibian artists. Black and white lino-cuts by one of our most famous artists, John Muafangejo, one of which depicts Peter and Bishop Colin Winter in the grounds of the Namibia Peace Centre outside Oxford. An abstract representation of an outsize zebra with small figures of other animals and hunters surrounding it, reminiscent of the San style of rock paintings. Photographs of dramatic rock formations. On the wall going up the stairs, I place a mixed media painting of the head and shoulders of a young black woman, who we call our African princess.

'I'm going to create a special corner under the stairs,' I tell Isabel.

I arrange Namibian baskets that belong to the embassy there, and water paintings I've brought with us that are illustrations of traditional folk tales I published at New Namibia Books. In one, a giant green snake emerges from a river with children in its mouth; in another, an *ekishi* monster creeps up behind a woman pounding maize; and in yet another, three Ovahimba children step out of broken ostrich eggs, illustrating a creation myth from the north-west of Namibia.

'It's beautiful Mummy,' Isabel tells me.

'Thank you, sweetheart,' I reply. 'I want to use the residence to showcase Namibian products.'

Allowance has been made in the embassy budget for two people to be employed at the residence: a cook and a housekeeper. The previous ambassador brought someone from Namibia to be his cook, but she has gone back home again. I've been making simple family meals since we arrived. If we want something more, we go out to one of the many good restaurants we are discovering around Brussels.

'I want us to get a cook,' Peter says to me.

'But I don't know how to work with a cook,' I respond. 'The thought terrifies me.'

'Why?'

'I don't know. Having to be responsible for thinking up meals. Telling someone what to do. Overseeing the whole process....' I falter.

'A cook would be there to help you,' Peter says. 'Not the other way around.'

I know we'll have to entertain at some point and a cook will be vital, but I'm still nervous about the idea. The embassy staff takes over, at Peter's instructions, and advertises and interviews people for the position.

'Do I get to meet this person before they're given the job?' I ask Peter.

'Don't worry, it'll work out alright,' he reassures me.

A young Filipino woman, Juliet, is appointed. She's dark-haired, petite, and works fast.

'Good morning, Madame,' she greets me cheerfully each day. 'What's for lunch today?'

Normally, I don't cook from menus and I don't plan meals before shopping; I buy what looks good that day or week and make meals from that. There's so much choice in Brussels, it's easy to work this way. When we first arrived, we were presented with too many choices in the supermarket: a whole aisle of mayonnaise and salad dressings, dozens of different types of coffee, large counters of cheeses, patés and saucisson. I've got used to it all now. The supermarket we usually go to has fresh fruit and vegetables and a large meat display. Rabbit, horsemeat, lark and other birds I've never eaten before, are stacked alongside the beef, lamb, chicken and pork I'm used to in Namibia.

I don't try these new meats but I continue to buy a range of other food and a lot of vegetables. So my answer to Juliet is,

'Let's see what's in the fridge.'

She takes out vegetables and prepares delicious soups. She makes meatballs, steaks, chips, potatoes au gratin Dauphinoise; all things I never do.

Juliet and I go together to the supermarket and she runs up and down the aisles, picking out new spices and ingredients. She critically examines the fruit and vegetables, chooses what is freshest, and suggests different cuts of meat. We progress to visiting the meat market where we buy in bulk at reduced prices, and the fruit and vegetable market, which has the freshest produce. She encourages me to go to the markets near our house on Wednesdays and Fridays, where there's organic produce

162

and locally made cheeses and jams. The meals she makes are to her own menus, varied, healthy and very good.

'What did we do without her?' I ask Peter, thinking of my former nervousness.

As I come to know her, I discover Juliet's story. She has two children, a son just older than Isabel and a daughter just younger, but she hasn't seen them for ten years. Her husband deserted the family, went to live in America, and started a new family there. Juliet left the Philippines in search of work to support her children and her mother, who looks after them. She learnt to cook in Singapore, before coming to Europe. She has outstayed her original visa and can't go home to visit her family because she wouldn't be able to come back.

'We're trying to help her regularise her status,' Peter reassures me.

As the diplomatic season starts up in late January, Peter and I are invited to the palace for the King and Queen's reception. The ambassadors and their spouses line up in strict order of seniority, according to when they presented their credentials. We wait in rooms with gilt pillars and vast chandeliers. There are footmen in frock coats everywhere. Our embassy officials tell me that since the Queen will be present, I must wear a dress or skirt, not trousers, and I've put on the outfit I bought for Peter's presentation of credentials. We file in, greet the King and Queen, shake their hands and extend our New Year greetings from our President, our country. Formal photos are taken with the King and Queen and we move on. We gather for refreshments in the Mirror Room. It has large gold maps of Africa above the doors, highlighting the Congo, and walls decorated in marble and copper. The ceiling and chandeliers are emerald green; they have been redone in recent years with the carapaces of more than a million jewel beetles.

Peter and I are invited to other receptions and I meet other wives of ambassadors. I begin to learn the protocol of diplomatic life, the forms of address, and the orders of seniority. I learn how to talk to people I know nothing about, whose views may differ widely from my own. I draw inspiration from memories of Deedee's courtesy, her openness and friendliness to all. I am more cautious than she is about expressing my opinions, not wanting to tread on any diplomatic toes, but I realise that I can always talk about Namibia, and I accept that as my role.

One day Peter comes home from the embassy looked very pleased.

'We're in luck,' he says. 'The Ministry of Foreign Affairs has agreed to cover the cost of renovations at the residence. Some other capital project fell through and they need to commit the funds to something else so the Ministry of Finance doesn't take it back. It's enough to cover all the renovations we need.'

The embassy gets quotations for the necessary work and chooses a contractor, a Flemish-speaking Belgian with whom I converse in stilted French when he comes to look at the house and measure up. The renovations will take three months, and we move into a small two-bedroom flat a few kilometres away while they are done. Mamadou takes me to the residence every other day to see how work is progressing. I used to be able to read French literature but I never learned the words for painting, tiling, mending doors, screws, etc. I start to acquire those now.

The flat is on the ground floor of a small three-storied block. Isabel and I almost prefer it to the residence, as we sit and talk together or I read while she does her homework, instead of being in different rooms, far apart. We have access to a tiny patch of garden, and we put up a washing line so we can dry clothes there. The neighbours knock on our door.

'*C'est interdit* – It's not allowed,' they tell us. No one seems to dry their laundry outside in Brussels.

There are other, higher apartment blocks behind ours, but we are at the end of the street and to one side there's a narrow lane and another field of mealies. We are near a tram stop, on a different line from our own, and I start to go in and out of town by myself. I enjoy the rhythm of the trams as they rock from side to side, passing behind gardens or along streets of brick terrace houses with large windows framed with flowers and plants. But I'm surprised at how diffident I feel to travel on my own, how dependent I've become through my months of sickness and the luxury of being driven around since we arrived in Brussels.

As part of the renovations, the residence will be painted and the builder gives me a colour pallet from which to choose. There's no money for new furnishings so the colours must fit what's already there. The rooms are large, the ceilings high, the windows and doors painted white. I choose strong colours to bring warmth to the residence: apricot beige for the reception rooms, with a lighter toning colour in the hall; crushed strawberry on two walls of our bedroom. I give Isabel free choice for her bedroom to make it feel more like her own, and she opts for a dark lilac.

One of the officers at the embassy worries about my choices and phones to consult the Ministry of Works in Windhoek about the colour code for diplomatic residences.

'You're only allowed three colours,' she reports to me. 'And they must all be pastel shades, so that nothing offends any future ambassador.'

'Oh,' I say in a non-committed way. I discuss it later with Peter.

'Don't take any notice,' he says.

'Perhaps I should tell them pastel colours offend me,' I joke.

I reduce the number of colours but hold onto the strongest, using Isabel's lilac for one of the guest bedrooms as well. We christen it the Jacaranda room.

We move back into the residence as spring comes. It's the briefest of seasons in Namibia. For 10-14 days in late August/early September, as soon as the night temperatures rise, and even without rain, the trees and thorn bushes begin to flower; the heady smell of jasmine fills the gardens. After that, it's just hot. In contrast, this is my first European spring in many years. I delight in the crocuses, in scarlet tulips, the greening of the weeping willow by the house and, in May, an explosion of rhododendrons in violet and crimson; by chance, they are the same colours I have used in the bedrooms.

With Juliet on board, the renovations finished and Isabel now settled at school, I decide it's time to improve my French. I've forgotten a lot and there are large holes in my vocabulary. I struggle to deal with many everyday situations such as the bank, the hairdresser or the gym we decide to join.

No one else in the family speaks French. Isabel is learning at school; Peter has little time for classes. So I have become the family facilitator, translating as much as I can in restaurants and receptions. I'm keen to improve, and I sign up for an intensive month-long course at a language school not far from the residence. Here I meet women from other countries who, like me, have come to Brussels for a while: Nita from Indonesia, Ana from Portugal, Maki and Naomi from Japan.

During the course, we revise the future tense.

'*Expliquez quelquechose que vous voudrez fair ou vous aller faire* – Talk about something you would like to do or are going to do,' the teacher tells us. '*On commence avec Nita.*'

Nita talks about her plans for a holiday at home in Indonesia. She and her husband Aachim will go to spend a week on Bali.

When it comes to me, I don't know what to say. There's nothing I have planned. I had hoped just to get to Brussels and to live. I don't know what the future holds and I am loath to start to dream of it.

I have no future and I don't know who I am. I feel that I've lost my professional life. I feel that I'm also losing the country I have come to call my own, my claim to be Namibian contradicted by my accent and appearance. Although I talk about Namibia and refer to it as home, I'm seen and heard by most people in Brussels as being English.

One day I open my emails and find one from a colleague who works in support of publishing in Africa.

'I've given your name to an NGO in The Netherlands. They're looking for someone to review the work of Femrite, the women's writers' association in Uganda,' it says.

They write to me the same week and ask for my CV. A few days later, they phone to discuss the possibility of me doing this consultancy. I tentatively agree and then discuss it with Peter.

'I want to try this,' I tell him. 'I haven't been anywhere on my own since I was ill, except to visit Doris and Clive in the Cape, so it feels like a big thing. But it's the sort of work I could still do from time to time here, and that would be good for me.'

'Do it,' he encourages me. 'Just don't overdo it.' I smile. It's a well-used Namibian expression.

The NGO asks me to go for three weeks but settles for two. I still don't have the energy I used to have before my heart collapsed and at times I get very tired, so I don't want to be away too long.

It's an interesting project within my knowledge and capabilities and, although I've heard about Femrite, I don't know it very well. It brings together women writers, runs workshops to help them develop their writing and publishes books written by its members. I'm interested in finding out more and wonder if a similar association could be set up to support women writers in Namibia.

I've visited Kampala before but only briefly, for an APNET conference. It's very different from Windhoek, much more tropical and with different colours – red earth, green trees and grey clouds. While I'm there this time, it's wet and cold some days, as we get the tail of a cyclone over Madagascar that sucks in the desert air from the Sahara and brings mist to the mountains of Uganda and Rwanda.

Kampala's infrastructure is poor, the buildings look old and dilapidated and the markets are full of stalls selling second-hand clothes from Europe – the country is slowly finding its way back from a succession of civil wars. I stay in a modest hotel that has dark wood paneling on the bedroom walls making the room gloomy, but I have a little desk to work at and look onto trees outside my window. I'm picked up from the hotel every morning by one of the women who work at Femrite, and she takes me to their office. When I go on from there to other meetings, another young woman writer takes me in a *matatu* – a kombi taxi full

167

of people. I'm the only white person. The other passengers look at me, shift up to give me space and continue with their conversations. My companion pays our fares and tells them when to stop. The *matatus* bounce uncomfortably across pot-holed roads, in great contrast to our smooth journeys in the chauffeur-driven Mercedes in Brussels.

The days are long and intense. I design a questionnaire for Femrite members, interview many of them and have meetings with other writers, booksellers, publishers, and NGOs in the book and educational sector. I go to Makerere University to interview a professor in the English Literature department.

'What difference has this association made to writers in Uganda?' I ask him.

'They're doing well,' he says. 'Really, they are the vanguard of a new renaissance of Ugandan writing.'

When I went to study at Sussex University in 1970, Makerere was a top African university, where ideas and writing flowed. Prominent African leaders and writers had studied there, including the Tanzanian President Julius Nyerere and the renowned Kenyan novelist Ngugi wa Thiong'o. The years after Idi Amin's takeover in Uganda in 1971 put paid to that. Hundreds of thousands of people were imprisoned and killed. Intellectuals fled the country. The civil war and unrest of the following two decades destroyed institutions and infrastructure. Today, Makerere is operating once again but it's a shadow of its former self. The buildings are old and in need of repair. Lecturers survive in small offices with little equipment.

'I can't overemphasise the importance of maintenance,' a Commonwealth university adviser told Peter when he was Vice Chancellor at the University of Namibia. But the finances are needed before maintenance work can be done, and a stable political and economic environment is needed to secure the financing.

The books published by Femrite are not light reading. They include novels, short stories and interviews with women, and deal with social and political issues. They tell of women's experiences within Ugandan society: physical abuse, rape, teenage pregnancy, forced marriage, women forced out of their homes when their husbands die.

I ask to visit schools that buy the books, and am taken to a top Catholic secondary school just outside Kampala and another school in the slum area of the city.

'Do you use these books in your teaching?' I ask.

'Yes, for literature and for social studies,' the teachers in both schools reply. 'The pupils really respond to these stories and that provides an opening to discuss many things. They see the stories as close to theirs and it helps to encourage them to write their own stories as well.'

In the evenings, I'm on my own. I write my notes on the day and read the 12 books and two magazines Femrite has published in the past five years. I'm pleased to have no other distractions so I can concentrate on the work, in contrast with previous consultancies I did in Namibia. There, I remember trying to run the family, home, publishing house and bookshop at the same time as doing consultancies, and the dreadful feeling I had of being torn in different directions. This time, Peter is returning earlier from the embassy to be with Isabel. Juliet has said she will prepare a snack for Isabel to come home to after school, and be with her for a while before she leaves to go home.

The trip is harder, though, than I imagine. I promise to present a draft of my findings before I leave but I'm trying to squeeze what was suggested as a three-week trip into two, so the pressure is on. One afternoon, as I drink sweet spiced tea with a publisher I'm interviewing, I feel a rapid run of extra heartbeats. My mouth goes dry and I feel dizzy.

'I'm sorry, but I don't feel very well,' I tell the publisher. 'I'd like to go back to the hotel and lie down.'

'I'll call a taxi,' he says. I wonder why I didn't plan transport by taxis for the work I've been doing, instead of criss-crossing town in *matatus*.

I can feel the extra heartbeats through that night and the next day and night. I don't know if it's the food or nerves or heart or heat or all of these, but I'm scared. They continue off and on until I get safely back to Brussels, when they stop.

I write up the final report on my return, falling into a narrative description that takes it to a 100 pages. I email Deedee to tell her about it and she laughs at me in her reply.

'You have to cut it down and write an executive summary as well, Jane, or no one will read it,' she writes.

I try to follow her advice and put sections in appendices as well but I find it hard to get away from the descriptions and just concentrate on analysis.

I take it easy for a month after the consultancy is over. Then, I turn to networks in Brussels set up for the international community, looking for friends and for things to do. I join Welcome to Belgium, a club run by wives of Belgian diplomats for spouses of ambassadors that organises various activities, including visits around the country. I also join the British and Commonwealth Women's Club (BCWC), which does similar things and provides a book club, exercise and arts groups. Their clubhouse is a two-storied terrace house in a residential area; it's a 15-minute walk from our house.

One of the women from BCWC takes me to join a small French/English conversation group, from two until four on Monday afternoons. We are ten women, half of us English-speaking, the other half French-speaking Belgians. We converse for an hour in French and an hour in English, each of us speaking about what we have been doing, or reading, or thinking, in the language we're trying to master. The English-speaking women are mostly middle-aged and are in Brussels because of their husbands' work, like I am. They stay until they're posted elsewhere. The Belgian women set up the group a decade ago; they're in their sixties and seventies. They tell us about changes in Brussels and in Belgian society and about the German occupation of Belgium during the Second World War.

We all take turns to host the conversation group in our sitting rooms, and provide tea and biscuits, prepared in advance and laid out on a table or a tray. At three o'clock, as we switch from one language to the other, the hostess goes to turn the kettle on and make the tea. We rise to collect our cups. The Belgian women all drink tea without milk, and without lemon as well. They choose delicate teas that taste delicious that way, not the strong black tea of England and Southern Africa that goes orange when milk is added. When the group comes to me, I give them Rooibos, the alternative tea of Southern Africa that has no caffeine, which is also best without milk.

Margaret talks about her son, who is a pilot in the British Royal Air Force, currently serving in Afghanistan.

'You know, he worked for a year at a school in the north of Namibia,' she tells me in English while we collect our tea one Monday, 'before he went to university. He loved it there. We went out to visit him.'

'Perhaps we met while you were there,' I say. 'Your face seems so familiar. When were you in Windhoek?'

'We didn't stay in Windhoek at all,' she says. 'We went straight to the north from the airport. But your face is familiar to me as well.' Each time we see each other, we try to find out if and where we might have met, but we can't pin it down.

Anne, one of the Belgians, tells us about her son's hot-air balloon – *une montgolfière*, it's called in French. He recently won an international ballooning competition. Carol, one of the English women, gives us detailed accounts of the hockey games she plays. I talk, as ever, about Namibia – *la Namibie*.

Haltingly, we discuss the recent mission to Titan (the moon of Saturn), the dalliances and illegitimate children of royal families in Britain, Belgium and The Netherlands, exhibitions at various art galleries and museums, amongst other things. I value the contact with women who have had different experiences from me and who are different from the people we meet more officially.

I also join the group of wives of ambassadors from Africa, the Caribbean and the Pacific (ACP). These countries come together as a bloc to negotiate on matters of trade with the European Union – the main focus for all our embassies. The ambassadors meet regularly and discuss existing and changing trade agreements. The spouses' group meets once a month at the home of a different member, in rotation. The meetings are informal, charity work is organised, but mostly the host introduces her country to the other members, offering traditional food, displaying crafts and information.

Thirty women from ACP countries gather for the first such meeting I attend, hosted by Tunisia. We all arrive by car, sweeping in convoy round the semi-circular drive, alighting at the door, while the drivers move on to return later at our bidding.

Despite the cold weather, some of the African women wear traditional, brightly coloured dresses with embroidered necks, cloths tied elaborately on their heads and shawls draped round their shoulders. Others are wearing Western clothes – trousers and skirts, jackets, sweaters. Most are smart but not ostentatious. I'm in dark red trousers made out of silk, from a tailored suit I had made in Namibia but have hardly worn before, with a black sweater and fine red and purple beads from Kenya.

I come at the appointed time and go round to those who are already there. Since I'm new to the group, I don't know most of the women and I try to gauge whether the person I'm introducing myself to is French- or English-speaking.

'*Bonjour, je m'appelle Jane. Je viens de la Namibie.*' We shake hands. I move on to the next person and the next, and then find a place to sit. The women are friendly, but they gather in groups of known friends, to some extent based on language and geography. When no one else sits by me, I move to join the wife of the Ambassador of Kenya, whom I've met before.

'How are you, Grace?' I ask.

'I'm well.'

'How are the children settling in?' She's also a recent arrival.

'They're doing well, thank you.'

My English upbringing taught me not to ask direct or personal questions, and I've never been good at social small talk. But I am learning now to start conversations by asking people about themselves: children, family, home, house, work. These are important to everyone, everywhere. I tell them about my family, and about Namibia.

I look round the room. It's one of three large reception rooms that lead off each other, with doors that can fold open and divide, or back to allow a big gathering. The walls are pale blue. The chairs and sofas are heavy and ornate and large mirrors in gold frames hang on the walls. Tunisian ornaments and boxes with beautiful inlaid decorations are scattered on low tables around the room. A woman moves quickly past us, dressed in turquoise trousers and a long tunic and disappears through a door. There are sounds from behind it of instruments being tuned.

We're treated to a performance from a Tunisian band – five men in traditional trousers, shirts and waistcoats, with modern and traditional instruments – a violin, hand-held drums, a lute and a Tunisian bagpipe.

'How is it made?' someone asks.

'It's a goatskin stretched and sewn into a bag. The pipes are attached to blow into and play on,' our hostess explains. Her name is Claude; she's a white Frenchwoman married to the Tunisian Ambassador.

The musician gives a short solo to demonstrate how the instrument works. The haunting sound takes me back to a collaborative musical performance I saw in Namibia last year, given by the university choir

172

together with a visiting Scottish choir. Three women – the keening angels of death – sang a lament while marching solemnly forward to claim those who had fallen in their journey of life. I remember thinking at the time that I wouldn't mind those women coming for me when my time is up – firm, strong and not to be argued with – women into whose care I would put my soul.

A belly dancer weaves her way into the room and dances as the Tunisian band start their performance. She ripples her body with a wry smile on her face. At first, the band plays soft music from one part of the country. Then the musicians pick up pace and the music becomes much more exuberant. The woman in turquoise, who we saw earlier, comes in to dance, stamping her feet to make the bells round her ankles sound, a long shawl tied round her hips with tassles that shake as she does. The intimacy of the dancing surprises me, my perception of Muslim societies so dominated by Islamic fundamentalism and the covering up and separation of women. However, I feel that we are somehow behind the veil now, in the private quarters of the women.

Claude brings in extra shawls and hands them round to members of the group so we can join in. All the Tunisian women do so immediately, as if they have been waiting for this opportunity to dance. Soon we are all there, in different groupings, coming and going, dancing together, learning new steps and inventing our own. We hold the shawls up above our heads, arms swaying while we make our way to the dance floor, or tie them round our hips like the dancer, to exaggerate our hip movements. This is a group to belong to, I think, diplomatic wives gathering together each month to dance!

Peter is also accredited to The Netherlands and to the Grand Duchy of Luxembourg. I accompany him when he presents his credentials to Queen Beatrix in The Hague and to the Grand Duke, head of state of Luxembourg, in the summer. For these formal occasions, I go shopping in search of a new outfit. I have already packed away my loose African dresses and the flat open sandals I used to wear in Namibia and have started to collect a new wardrobe for my role as ambassador's wife: smart trousers and skirts, little jackets, and enclosed shoes with low heels. Now I need something lighter as the weather is warmer.

I find a smart red and cream dress with matching cream jacket, shoes and bag. The dress needs altering to fit, as the top is too big for me. When it's ready, I ask Mamadou to take me to the store to collect everything. On the way home he asks:

'Have you bought a hat, Madame?'

I shake my head, 'No.'

Mamadou pauses. 'The wife of the former Ambassador always wore a hat when she went to visit the Queen of The Netherlands,' he tells me gently. I go back to the shop to buy a matching hat as well.

In The Hague we're picked up from our hotel by a horse-drawn carriage and driven through the park to the Queen's palace. A footman stands at the back of the carriage as we ride and climbs down to assist us when we enter or leave it. We drive through the park and people wave at us; I don't know if we're supposed to wave back. A red carpet leads from the gates of the palace to its huge doors, and Peter has to inspect the guard of honour lined up alongside. I am allowed to join Peter for a conversation with the Queen.

The Netherlands has long been a partner of Namibia's. Dutch Government agencies and NGOs, political parties and trade unions supported the movement for independence and the development work of the new Government after 1990. The Queen has been well briefed on developments since Independence and asks detailed questions.

In Luxembourg, after Peter has presented his credentials to the Grand Duke, I join them for a photo call. We go on to have lunch with the Director of the Luxembourg Development Agency, LuxDev, which gives support to Namibia. We talk about the projects they are assisting that concentrate on integrated rural and urban development in the Kavango region in the north-east of the country. Sandy's husband Ted, a town planner, is working with them.

Peter is used to networking and discussing Namibia's development with top officials and politicians, to mixing with Heads of Government and Heads of State. I am not; it is a whole new world for me. Nor am I used to being fussed over, looked after, driven around, and addressed as 'Madame' by domestic and embassy staff. 'Madame' is less strange in the French-speaking environment of Brussels, since all married women are addressed this way, but it still takes some getting used to.

Claude, the wife of the Tunisian Ambassador, puts my name forward to replace her as a representative from Africa in the International Group of Ambassadrices, as she will be leaving Brussels soon. This group has some 20 members representing different regions and continents. It also meets once a month, arranging more formal sit-down lunches for their members, with a short cultural show, food from the host's country, and gifts for all the guests. The irony is not lost on me of a white European wife of an African ambassador recommending another white European wife to represent the African continent. But it's good for Namibia and for me, and I tell them that I'm interested.

The chairperson of the group is Princess Margaret of Liechtenstein. She's the sister of the Grand Duke of Luxembourg, married to Prince Nicholas of Liechtenstein, who is his country's Ambassador in Belgium. She arranges to come to our residence to meet me before confirming my membership of the group.

'The house must look immaculate,' I tell Concepcion beforehand. 'She's a princess.'

'Please, have tea and coffee and juice ready,' I say to Juliet. 'And can you make some of those lovely Swedish biscuits you do?'

I buy flowers and put them in the sitting room. I fuss about the arrangement of the ornaments and check that the guest toilet is clean and the towel is fresh.

When the princess arrives, I take her into the large sitting room. She is friendly, gracious and informal, dressed in dark trousers and a blouse.

'Can I offer you something to drink?' I ask her.

'No thank you,' she replies.

'Please, just a cup of tea or coffee?'

'No thank you,' she says again.

'Some juice perhaps?'

'Alright, yes, some orange juice please.'

In this way, I force something on her. When I think about it after she has gone, I feel embarrassed. But the rest of the conversation goes well and the princess formally invites me to join the group.

When it's my turn to host a luncheon, I think about what to do for the 'cultural' component and decide I want to show a film about Namibia. I look through the videos and DVDs at the embassy; they are geared towards tourists and show landscapes, deserts and animals, but hardly any people. I have problems with these representations of Namibia. With only two million of us in a country that's twice the size of Germany, the population density is very low but it's the capital, the other towns, the communal rural areas and the farms that hold the real life of Namibia – its people.

I decide instead to put together an exhibition on the lives of women in Namibia. I go through all our books, magazines and tourist brochures – our own and those at the embassy. I cut and copy, print out captions and mount them on freestanding display boards I get the embassy to buy. It's a real old-fashioned scissors and paste job of which I am well pleased. I place woven baskets, embroidered cloths, carved animals and other crafts on tables, jewellery I have that is made from ostrich eggshells or porcupine quills, and books by Namibian women writers that I've brought from home. The photos concentrate on women in the rural areas – milking, cultivating, pounding millet, making pots, and sewing. I make sure there are also urban or 'modern' images – women at a soccer match drinking beer, women science students at the university, models in leather or fur coats made in Windhoek, Miss Namibia contestants and photos of leading women in public life – the Attorney General, the Minister of Home Affairs, the Minister of Finance, the Deputy Prime Minister, and the Managing Director of the diamond company NAMDEB.

I hire large round tables and chairs for the day, and Juliet helps me arrange and decorate the room, as well as preparing the food. Mamadou and Pascal guide the cars and their drivers as they drop the wives of the ambassadors. Concepcion has donned a black dress and serves drinks to people as they arrive – sparkling wine and juice – on silver trays. The cook from the residence of the Embassy of Barbados and one of her friends help to serve as well.

As the guests arrive, they take a drink and are guided into one of our linked reception rooms (we normally use it as a family TV room but it's been cleared and decorated for the day). After everyone has gathered there, I play a five-minute video of Namibia, showing the desert, animals and other tourist delights, while the display boards are put into place in the entrance hall.

I take a sip from my glass of champagne, and start to speak.

'*Princesse, chères soeurs, fellow ambassadrices, soyez bien-venues.* Welcome to Namibia. *Je suis tres contente de vous recevoir aujourd'hui. Nous avons preparer la nourriture Namibienne pour vous, mais avant le repas il y a une esposition sur la vie des femmes en Namibie.*' I indicate that they may move back to the entrance hall. '*Je vous en prie.*'

The women walk in and around the display, looking at photos, picking up pieces of jewellery and talking to each other.

'*Mais c'est tres jolie* – it's very pretty,' one says as she looks at a necklace made of porcupine quills.

'What is this for?' another asks, pointing to a large woven basket with handles and a narrow neck plugged with a piece of wood.

'It's from the north of Namibia,' I reply. 'It's used for making butter. You put the milk in and then shake it until it turns into butter.'

'Hard work, I think,' the woman says.

'Yes.'

'Why do you only have photos of tribal women?' one of the European ambassadrices asks, and I realise there is only one white face in my display – a young German-speaking woman who was Miss Namibia a couple of years ago. I don't want to deal head-on with the racist implications of her comment.

'I worked with the images that were available,' I tell her, but I think I should have found a better reply.

My parents are with us. They've come to stay for two weeks and I ask them to join us for lunch. Normally, our luncheons are women only, and my father is the only man to eat with us today. I didn't want to ask if it would be alright, because I didn't want to give anyone the opportunity to say no. He looks quite happy, sipping champagne, surrounded by elegant women, a little smile beneath his moustache.

'I wish my parents were so close they could come to visit,' says the wife of the Ambassador of Singapore.

The tables are not red this time, but large and round, covered with white tablecloths. The crockery is gold-rimmed with the national emblem of Namibia printed on it. We savour beef from Namibia and poached cod – one of the main types of fish Namibia has, although in this case it's not from Namibian waters. The entrée is smoked game salami salad – the game salami brought over by Peter in his suitcase after a recent trip to a Foreign Ministry meeting back home. Deedee chose the gifts – linen cushion covers hand-embroidered by members of a women's cooperative – and sent them to me via Peter.

So I learn to entertain. I give ladies' lunches and teas. We invite people for dinner. We hold receptions at the residence and elsewhere. We entertain visiting groups of students and the alumni in Belgium of St Antony's College, Oxford, where Peter did his DPhil in the 1980s. As long as I have enough time to plan it all, I don't mind, but I find it hard when something is arranged at short notice by the embassy. In either case, Juliet holds it all together. She knows how to prepare and present the food and lay the tables beautifully. We borrow ideas from other embassy staff or their spouses about Namibian dishes we can present. However much I claim to be Namibian, my culinary skills and knowledge were developed elsewhere, so providing a 'Namibian meal' has been a challenge.

How to represent Namibia is an issue that concerns me. Do I focus on the beauty of the land, where there are so many wonderful animals in the wild? The cheetah capital of the world, with more cheetahs than any other country and the headquarters of the Cheetah Conservation Fund? More elephants than we can cope with – many in the Etosha reserve but also problem ones that trample crops and damage houses, especially in Caprivi. There are also elephants in the Namib – a living desert with specially adapted animals, and lions that come down to the sea.

Do I talk about political stability, about our growing culture of parliamentary democracy, enshrined in the Constitution and led in the National Assembly by the Speaker, our friend Mosé Tjitendero? Do I acknowledge that the democratic practices still need to be strengthened at regional and party level? It's a country where a high percentage of the budget is spent on health and education, where the literacy rate has gone up from 60 to 80 per cent since Independence, although there are still many children who leave school without the skills to get a job.

Namibia is a land rich in natural resources – diamonds, uranium, zinc, copper, fish, and beef, with a good telecommunications and transport infrastructure; very attractive for investors. A land with excellent private health clinics, private schools and a First-World standard of living for those who have the money. Yet whites still own the majority of the land utilisable for agriculture and still control large sectors of the economy. It's a land where too often white people still employ family members rather than advertise for the best qualified, and black economic empowerment empowers very few.

Do I talk about a land where many people still live in poverty, with one of the highest income differentials in the world? There are people with so much money, acquired before Independence or afterwards. Then there are those, like Peter's younger brother David, who live on the meagre proceeds of semi-precious stones scraped from the desert with their bare hands. And pastoralists in the south of the country whose sheep must eat rocks because nothing seems to grow there. We have one of the most unequal societies in the world, yet we are still rated as one of Africa's success stories. One reason for our success is that the black middle class is growing and staying at home because life is good there, and their professional and technical skills help to keep the economy growing. It is a land where the rate of infection with HIV/AIDS is one of the five highest in the world, where racism persists, sexism is deep in all communities and domestic violence is all too common. These are the challenges we face.

As an embassy, we must stress the positive. Nevertheless, one day I can be talking about tourism and investment opportunities and the next day about the sexual behaviour of our countrymen and women, with reference to the high incidence of HIV/AIDS.

The demands of Peter's work negotiating with the European Union for better access to its market for Namibian goods, or with the World Trade Organisation in Geneva that we also cover, take precedence over bilateral relations with Belgium, Luxembourg and The Netherlands. Peter and I get too few opportunities to meet people from these countries and move mostly in the international circles of Brussels. Most of the people Peter works with are from the African, Caribbean and Pacific (ACP) countries and the European Union. Most of the women I know come from the ACP or other non-European countries.

The people who work with us are also from other parts of the world. Juliet and Concepcion are Filipino, while Mamadou comes from Senegal and Pascal from Benin. At the embassy, apart from the Namibian diplomats, the locally recruited staff members come from other African countries, with one from France; there are no Belgians. In this way, we are introduced to the network of immigrant workers who serve so many embassies and form the core of staff at diplomatic residences. The stories, like Juliet's, of how they came to Europe and found work, move and amaze me. I'm impressed at the way they send remittances to families at home, whose fortunes they have to follow at a distance of geography and time.

There's widespread prejudice in Europe against immigrants, however, and between different language and religious groups. In Belgium, there is institutionalised separation of the Flemish and French communities. The country is divided into Flemish, French and German regions with wide-ranging powers that include education. The German region, in the east, is small and ignored by the other two, who compete with each other for national dominance. Different districts, or communes, in Brussels are administered by Flemish or French officials, based on the number of mother-tongue speakers of one or the other language registered as residents within the commune. All documentation from the commune is in the language of the dominant group. Belgian politicians make openly hostile public comments about members of the other group, as do individual citizens.

This is the sort of segregation that has blighted southern Africa, and it shocks me to see it here. With Namibia's Independence and the coming of democracy and non-racial government to South Africa, divisions between people on the basis of language, race or community are no longer accepted. However imperfect we are at achieving it in practice, most people in southern Africa agree that we must try to respect each other and work together.

Earlier this year, in May 2004, the European Union's latest expansion took in ten new members, mostly from the former Eastern bloc. The centre of Brussels was full of dark blue EU flags, with a central circle of gold stars, fluttering in celebration. People from the new member states spoke positively about joining the EU.

'It's only now that the Second World War has finally ended,' the wife of the Czech Ambassador told me at the luncheon she gave for the International Ambassadrices Group. I hadn't thought of it like that.

Some of the older EU countries were fearful that workers from these new member states would swamp them. Most imposed restrictions on the number of workers they would allow in, but this does not stop talk in the media and at private dinner tables about Polish plumbers and builders taking over.

One of the teams of builders who worked on our renovations for the residence was Polish; the other was Belgian. The Poles quoted a lower rate for the work they did on the annexe flat. They came at seven in the morning and worked until six at night, and on Saturdays as well. The Belgians came at nine in the morning and worked until four, and never at the weekend.

There is particular prejudice in Belgium and other parts of Europe against Muslims and fear about Islamic fundamentalism. But, for me, this time in Brussels is a period of discovery. I am learning about other religions and cultures, including Islam; learning to respect, not just accept, them. Through the women's groups, I come to know the rhythms of the Muslim faith – the time for prayer, the Friday mosque, the calendar of festivals, the fasting month of Ramadan and the delicious dates eaten as darkness falls, to break the fast.

Through long discussions in the car with our Muslim driver, Mamadou, I come to appreciate his sense of justice and his compassion. I come to appreciate the expression 'Insha'Allah' – God willing – because I know now that I cannot control the future.

The journeys in the car become discussion forums as we drive to meetings, to the shops, to neighbouring towns, listening on the way to the BBC World Service. The news is dominated by Iraq. I've tried to shut it out since early 2003, at the time that I became so ill, when it became clear that the USA and UK were going to invade without the backing of the UN. The celebratory TV images of tanks rolling towards Baghdad were too much for me to take. So too, the news of developments since then as Iraq has descended into an ongoing war of attrition between the occupying forces and those who oppose them.

But I am beginning to take my head out of the sand. More than a year after the invasion of Iraq, I attend a public tribunal on the war, held in a hotel in central Brussels. It's one of a series of meetings held around the world, structured as a commission of inquiry into the war and the thinking behind it.

Mamadou drops me at the hotel. There's a large sign indicating that the tribunal is being held on the first floor. I walk up wide stairs with brass banisters and turn into a reception area filled with tables carrying information about Iraq: the war, the position of women there, what different groups are trying to do to mobilise international action against the war. I look briefly at a large display of photographs of damaged buildings and overcrowded hospitals in Baghdad. I turn into the main room where the tribunal is being held. The carpet is soft and dark red. A central table has been placed at the top of the room for the chairperson and commissioners of the tribunal. Tables for opposing defence and prosecution teams face each other, one on the left side of the hall and the other on the right. Dining chairs have been laid out in rows for the audience.

The tribunal is conducted along the lines of the Bertrand Russell Tribunals of 1967, which investigated war crimes committed during the Vietnam War. It is presided over by Father François Houtart, Professor Emeritus at the Catholic University of Louvain (in Belgium). His name is immediately familiar to me but I can't place it.

'Tell me who Father Houtart is,' I say to Peter when I go home at the end of the first day. 'He's chairing this tribunal.'

Peter smiles. 'Ah, so he's still busy. Good.' Then he tells me: 'Father Houtart chaired the first International Conference on Namibia held in Brussels in 1972.'

'The one you and Uazuvara were involved with?' I ask. I've heard stories about it before.

'Yes,' Peter goes on. 'The conference was organised by a national committee of political parties, trade unions and solidarity groups, in conjunction with SWAPO. Uazuvara was SWAPO Deputy Secretary for Foreign Affairs then. He was sent by SWAPO as our coordinator for the conference and I was assigned to assist him.'

'Wasn't he sick or something?' I ask.

'Yes. He got malaria and had a terrible fever. He spent days in bed. I drafted letters about the conference and signed them. Then I picked up his hand and got him to sign them as well – they were supposed to be signed by the two of us.'

At the tribunal, the defence and prosecution teams make opening and closing speeches. Witnesses, including academics, lawyers, political activists, NGOs and church groups, give testimony and are cross-examined. They talk about oil pipelines from Iraq to Europe, strategic geopolitical interests, the Project for the New American Century (PNAC) – the think-tank behind the Bush administration and its aggressive international stance. We're given information about the rise of these neo-conservatives in the USA and how some liberals, such as the UK Prime Minister Tony Blair, accepted their view of international intervention.

Iraqi men and women talk about the situation in the country that has already been devastated by the years of UN sanctions against the regime of Saddam Hussein. They cite the high rates of child mortality because of limited access to medicine. We hear more about the protests across the world in early 2003 in the attempt to stop US armed intervention. I pick up a leaflet about the Lysistrata Project of that time, when the same play that Sandy produced in 2001 in Namibia was performed in different countries as the focus of a peace initiative against war with Iraq.

My mind is stimulated by the information and the discussions, and all my old political instincts are revived. Life in Namibia has been strangely apolitical. I've been preoccupied with family life, raising children, running a business, involvement in networks supporting publishing in Africa; I haven't been politically active. The reigning political philosophy in Namibia since Independence has been 'pragmatism' – building bridges (between people and across dry riverbeds that flood dangerously in the rainy season), building the economy, developing health and educational services and access to them. There's been little political debate about ways of doing these things. Some of this is due to the push for national reconstruction after Independence. Some of it's to do with world politics. With the fall of the Soviet Union and the communist bloc, there's been

183

a dearth of ideological debate. We no longer know what socialism is or was meant to be, because of the collapse of the countries that called themselves socialist. We no longer know what alternatives there are to the neo-conservative ideologies that have dominated Western political thought since the early 1980s.

I want to share what I have heard, and I write a report about the tribunal afterwards. I give copies to the officers at the embassy, and send one home to the Foreign Ministry. No one responds or comments. I'd like to discuss it more widely with other diplomats in Brussels, but I don't know what their views might be, so I don't. That side of things is Peter's job, not mine. I also find it difficult to share this with other diplomatic spouses. Our conversations are blander, geared to what are considered women's issues – families, clothes, food and culture.

Brussels calls itself the capital of Europe and it does feel like the centre, not just because of the European Union headquarters but also because it offers great possibilities of travel. With the opening of borders between EU member states, passports are no longer needed; with the common monetary area, Euros can be used in most EU member states. The distances are also small. In two and a half hours – less time than it takes to drive from Windhoek to the sea – we can reach five other countries: Germany, The Netherlands, France, Luxembourg and England. We climb on the Eurostar, the high-speed train that connects Brussels with London, which hurtles through Belgium and France, into the tunnel that goes under the Channel, and we emerge in the gentle scenery of Kent. It's very different from the slow ferry crossings that were necessary when I last made this trip 30 years ago.

I'm able to see my parents more often, and to get closer once again to my English family, whom I've only seen on visits every year or two since we left Oxford 17 years ago.

'Jane is always trying to escape the English middle class,' a friend of mine used to say, as I searched for my own meaning when I was a young woman. But I see now that what I thought was an archetypically English middle-class family reflects both the liberal tradition of service and the changes in British society.

'You've all done different things,' my mother said to me when she and my father were with us in Windhoek after I was ill. 'John used to say that when you all grew up he wanted a doctor, a lawyer, an accountant and a plumber. But you've done things we wouldn't have expected. We're proud of you all.'

My parents, siblings and our children have gathered as a family when we could, the last occasion being to celebrate our parents' 50th wedding anniversary in 1998. We had a lunch together at a hotel near my parents' home, with other family members as well.

The hotel was a former private home, a rectangular Georgian-style building with tall windows and long lawns stretching from the front terrace. Many of us stayed there overnight and we stayed on in the UK for a week afterwards as well. Peter was in Canada for the annual meeting of Vice-Chancellors of the Association of Commonwealth Universities. He flew in the morning of the lunch and got a taxi from the airport directly to the hotel. He showered immediately after arriving and changed into a cream suit with a high-buttoned Nehru collar. I also wore a cream, trouser suit, made out of heavy silk, with a tie belt. I had coloured my hair an auburn red and had new gold-rimmed glasses.

'Interesting specs, Jane,' one of my cousins said to me at the lunch. 'You still in your Trotskyist stage?'

I laughed: 'These are the post-Trotskyist ones.' Although they were round, they had an extra line of metal that curled over the top of each lens, adding what I thought was a stylish flair.

We took a lot of photos. In one, my parents posed in a line with their eleven grandchildren, all of them with their hands on each other's shoulders, looking as if they were about to break into a dance. Their hair colours ranged from dark brown to red and blonde; the styles from a crew-cut to almost waist-length; short, wavy, thick, curly and straight. Their skin colours ranged from shades of white and cream to brown.

My younger sister, Helen's husband is Colombian. Rafael speaks to their sons in Spanish and Helen speaks to them in English; their accents are slightly Spanish and slightly American, from the international schools they've attended. Sarah's children grew up in Liverpool and have Liverpudlian accents. My brother John's have slight London accents. Perivi and Isabel's vowels and turns of phrase are southern African.

'It's so nice to hear the kids chatting to each other,' I said to Helen at the end of the day. 'I like the mixture of accents.' They are all in contrast to our parents' moulded BBC tones.

Now, in September 2004, we gather again for the wedding in England of John's daughter Beth. Peter, Isabel and I travel over to London on the Eurostar. Perivi is busy with his studies in Syracuse.

The ceremony and reception are held in the church run by John for over 20 years, in which his wife Anne and their children Abi, Beth, David and Simon, are all active. The church is full, the music is modern and the mood lively. We have champagne in the church grounds afterwards while chairs are moved, drapes are hung, and the church is transformed for the reception. A buffet meal is followed by a *ceilidh* – Scottish dancing. I join in for one or two reels but don't want to do too much. Peter, who has learnt Scottish dancing from Tricia and Richard in Namibia, continues long after me.

'*Ceilidhs* are traditionally connected with courting and marriage,' Anne tells me, and they're becoming really popular again.'

While Peter dances, I sit with Helen and we try to catch up with each others' news. It's six years since we saw each other. Helen has made her life in South and Central America, moving from one country to another, working with governments on environmental projects to protect bio-diversity. She is living and working now in Mexico but she started off in Brasil, doing research for her PhD when she was 22.

'Portuguese is just a mixture of French and Latin, both of which I know,' she told the scholarship body she had applied to for sponsorship of her PhD, 'and I feel confident I can pick it up quickly.' She did learn it, but it was harder than she expected. She was immersed immediately in the language when she went to Brasilia and stayed in a women's hostel there; no one else spoke English.

She met, Rafael, who is also an ecologist, during her fieldwork.

'I was in the Amazon forest, looking for birds,' Rafael likes to say, 'and I found Helen.'

They started their married life in Brasil but moved soon afterwards to Bogota, where Helen became fluent in Spanish as well. My parents went to evening classes and learnt Spanish to be able to speak to Rafael. They used it when they went to Bogota and met his family, and became fluent enough to read novels by the famous Colombian writer Gabriel Garcia Marquez in the original Spanish. I learnt some Spanish as well, but Rafael has mastered English now, and I've hardly ever used it.

'You're looking *muy elegante*,' I say to Helen now. I've dressed smartly, by happenchance in another cream suit, this time with a skirt, not trousers, and I wore a hard-brimmed beige straw hat in the church. But Helen is elegant in an un-English way. Her fingernails and toenails are varnished. Her little black shoes are strapless. She wears a black sleeveless chiffon dress with a beige pattern, and a twisted necklace and matching bracelet of silver and tiger's eye.

'I love your necklace, Helen,' I tell her. 'Tiger's eye is my favourite stone.'

'You always loved it,' she says. 'Do you remember you used to have a tiger's eye bracelet when you were about 12?'

'And I foolishly wore it while walking on the moors, and lost it,' I add.

Helen and I were very close as children. We were the 'little ones' and did a lot together. After she went to live in South America, we used to correspond by letter. Airmail envelopes came from Brasil with yellow and blue stripes round the edge and an array of beautiful stamps. Later, we sent each other long faxes, and later still, emails. Now, we communicate rarely. We both became preoccupied with our work and families, and she is always on the move, travelling to different countries, finishing a report or preparing for another trip.

'How's it all going, Helen?' I ask.

'I'm tired,' she says.

'Be careful,' I tell her. I've always felt protective of her. 'I think stress and exhaustion were factors in my heart collapsing the way it did.'

'I thought it was a virus,' she says.

'Yes, but you're more susceptible to viruses when you're severely run down.'

'Well, I'm lucky to have a big sis who I always come running to for comfort and advice. I still feel that even though you're miles away,' she tells me.

'Thanks,' I say, and then ask after her sons. 'How are Antonio and Danny?'

'They're well, but I'm sad they couldn't come,' she replies. 'Antonio's working on a television programme in Los Angeles since he completed his film degree, and Daniel's now in his second year of Finance and Film.'

'How does he find Chicago?' I ask.

'Cold, I think,' she says and laughs.

After breakfast together the next morning in the bed and breakfast we all stay in, Helen presents me with the tiger's eye necklace and bracelet.

'I want you to have them, Janie,' she says.

'Thank you so much, my dear! They're beautiful!' I respond.

In addition to reconnecting with family, I look up two old friends from my school days, Elizabeth and Susan. They've both visited us in Namibia, but we only see each other after intervals of many years.

Susan was my best friend in my first years of secondary school. We both dreamed of being doctors, or writers. She did study medicine but she found it hard seeing people die, and she moved into pathology instead. Tall, thin, with long, thick, sandy coloured hair, she still looks exactly like she did all those years ago.

Elizabeth joined the police after going to Oxford and rose through the ranks to become Britain's second woman chief constable, in charge of one of the counties. She's practical, perceptive, tough when she needs to be, but remarkably unhardened by her work.

They suggest meeting up with other friends from school whom I haven't seen for 20 years or more and Sue organises a lunch in London during one of my visits there. She chooses a little restaurant in Covent Garden.

It's Isabel's half-term holiday from school and she comes with me. We overnight with Sue at her house near Waterloo and walk with her to the restaurant the next day, across Waterloo Bridge. We pause on the bridge for Isabel to take photos of the panoramic view of London it affords, sweeping up the River Thames to the high-rise buildings of the financial centre in the City in the east, adjacent to the dome of St Paul's Cathedral, and in the other direction, towards the Houses of Parliament and the London Eye, the big, slow-moving Ferris wheel on the south bank of the river, built to celebrate the millennium.

'It's a pity that Liz couldn't come in the end,' Sue says, 'but nice that Gill and Linda can.'

'I haven't seen Linda since Perivi was two, and Gill since forever,' I tell her.

The five of us were a close group in our last year at school. We opened a shop for two weeks after our A-levels exams, cleaned and painted it, collected second-hand clothes and sold them to raise money for charity. We stayed for those two weeks in a little cottage on the outskirts of Leeds that belonged to Elizabeth's parents. Then we went on to different universities and grew apart.

When we get to the restaurant, Gill and Linda are already there and they get up when we come in, to greet and hug us. Linda's irrepressible giggle and big smile are immediately familiar from the past. Gill looks very much the same, her green eyes still intense and her dark brown hair still wavy, although it's shorter than when I saw her last.

The four of us order salads. Linda and I have glasses of dry white wine; Sue and Gill take water. Isabel orders a pizza and hot chocolate, but she doesn't like her drink when it comes; it's made the French way, by pouring boiling milk over solid blocks of chocolate that then melt.

'It's too strong,' she says. 'I'll just have some water.'

She sits at one end of the table and watches us with interest as the four of us ask each other questions about jobs, work and children. There's a lot of catching up to do.

'Well, I'm still doing pharmacy,' Linda tells me. 'Teaching at university and writing, still busy.'

'And you Gill?' She went to Cambridge and I always thought she'd be a writer.

'I'm teaching English to speakers of other languages,' she says, 'at a college in London.'

'Married?' I ask.

'Yes, to an architect, and we have one son.'

When I last met Gill I was in my late twenties and working with Peter in the SWAPO Office in London.

'Well, I married the boss,' I tell her, laughing, and try to give her a rundown of my life since then.

Linda, Sue and I last met as a group together, with Liz, when we were in our early thirties and preoccupied with establishing our own professional and family lives. The differences between what we were doing seemed more marked then. Now that we are older, the differences seem less.

'I think we all look the same as we did when we were 18,' I tell them. 'We might look a bit older but the hairstyles have hardly changed!'

The mannerisms of the past are still there. The personalities shine through the public faces we present, the professions we talk about, the family news. I'm reminded of how strong the essence of a person is. We think we grow and change but the core remains the same.

Just two hours drive east from Brussels, in northern Germany, Luther is closer to us than he's ever been before and he comes to visit. The first time, we sit on the leather sofas in the smart reception room, and he talks about how hard he has found life without Brigitte, how desperate he has felt in the apartment, alone.

'I couldn't stand it in the flat without Brigitte,' he says. 'I went out all the time to visit other people. I went to see Brigitte's parents downstairs every day. I walked round town. Anything except sitting in the apartment, with all the reminders of her.'

'Do they offer any grief counselling or support after you lose someone so close to you to cancer?' I ask him.

'There were some meetings I went to,' he replies, 'for people who'd lost their loved ones. They were good. I found it helpful just to talk and tell people what I was feeling.' He pauses. 'But, the people weren't there when I got home and shut the door.'

Two months later, Luther tells Peter quietly on the phone that he has met someone new.

'She lives nearby,' he said. 'I met her during my walks and we started talking.'

He arranges to bring her to meet us. I'm pleased for him but nervous; she too. When we meet, though, there is an easy acceptance of each other. She's different from Brigitte, slighter, less assertive, and with wavy brown, collar-length hair. She comes from the former East Germany, and has only lived in the west for the past year, having moved to Bochum when her son won a sponsored place in a technical college there. She looks lovingly at Luther when he speaks.

Peter's and my German is very limited, so we talk English and she tries to keep up with our chatter. The jokes are the same ones we're used to making with Luther and Brigitte, as if Brigitte were still here. For the first time in the two years since Brigitte died, Luther looks relaxed. But we have to remember that the name of the woman at his side is Evelin, that she doesn't share all the old familiar references. It must be hard for her, I think, following in the footsteps of someone who was so loved.

While Evelin takes a shower the following morning, Luther sits and chats to us at the table in the small breakfast room. He tells us that Brigitte's son Tobi urged him to speak to her father about Evelin.

'Tobi organised a sauna for the three of us,' Luther tells us. 'And when we were sitting there, he looked at me and said, "Go on, talk." So I told Papa Muller and he was very understanding.'

'What did he say?' I ask.

'He said "Life goes on, Luther. We know how much you loved Brigitte, but you must carry on living."'

'What about Brigitte's mother?' I want to know. 'How did she take it?'

'Mutti was silent when she heard the news,' Luther says. 'But some time later she gave Evelin a key to the front door of the apartment block. "You'd better have this so you can come and go more easily," she said to Evelin.'

Before Brigitte died, Luther promised her that he would look after her parents and now he stays in Germany to do so. He no longer refers to them as his in-laws but as his parents, too. The conflict they used to have evaporated when they came together to care for Brigitte in her last years. Now Evelin goes to visit them if Luther is away and increasingly they rely on her as well. I can't help thinking that somehow she was sent by Brigitte.

Norway is not easily accessible to us by train or by road, but it's a short flight away. We take advantage of this to visit Patji and Heidi. Peter, Isabel and I fly direct to Oslo and get the train into the city. We are under instructions to get off at a suburban station and Patji's mother Kirsten meets us there. She takes us over the road to a nearby bus stop from where we will continue. We catch up with each other's news until the bus arrives half an hour later. It's a 30-seater coach. We stow our luggage in the trunks at the side, climb on and pay the driver.

The bus route goes from Oslo to a number of little towns on the way to Skien, in southern Norway, where Patji and Heidi are now based, and then on further from there as well.

I turn to Peter. 'Can you imagine having a service like this in Namibia?' I ask. 'Wouldn't it be fantastic?'

'It's a far cry from the overcrowded buses that go from Windhoek to the north at weekends,' he says. 'Do you remember when Patji went up to Onandjokwe on one of those buses?'

'Yes. He didn't enjoy it much, though.'

The journey takes us two and a half hours. We go through tunnels as we leave Oslo, past farms, up steep hills as the road ascends over the mountains, and through pine forests. We see little villages and towns but, like Namibia, Norway is a large country with a small population, so there are large areas that look uninhabited.

Patji is completing his specialisation in obstetrics/gynaecology and working long hours at the local hospital in Skien. He and Heidi have a second child, a little girl called Meri, who is ten months old and already walking. Egil is now three. Heidi has just started working a few hours a week in a dress shop in town.

'I quite like it, you know,' she tells me when I ask about it. 'It gets me out of the house for a few hours and it's a good way of learning Norwegian. I need that before I can apply for something more in my line.' She has a Masters degree in Communication and worked with UNICEF when she was in Namibia. She already speaks Finnish, Swedish, English and German, so I have no doubt she will pick up Norwegian quickly.

They live in a small flat near the hospital, and Patji can walk to work. They have booked rooms for us in a little wood-board hotel surrounded by trees, that is also within walking distance from them. Isabel has to spend much of the time holed up at the hotel completing school projects, even though it's her half-term. Patji takes Peter and me out for a walk in the forest one morning. He carries Meri in a backpack. Egil is walking by himself.

'I'll just take it slowly,' I say to them. 'Go on ahead if you need to. I don't like hills.'

'How is your heart?' Patji asks me.

'It's fairly stable at the moment, with the pacemaker and the medicine I take,' I reply. 'But I can't do hills. My legs don't seem to move and my chest feels tight. So I'll walk a bit and rest a bit.'

'Doesn't the pacemaker speed up if you're doing exercise?' he asks.

'Yes, but not enough for hills apparently!'

'Does it just work when your heart needs it?'

'Well, I've seen a cardiologist in Brussels a couple of times, just for check-ups. He says my heart's completely dependent on the pacemaker now.'

I turn to see how Egil is doing. He's standing at the side of the path with a little stick, poking gently at something on the ground. I go to join him and bend down to look. It's a line of ants.

'Look at how they're carrying things,' I point out to him. 'See that one with a bit of leaf? Ants work hard, you know.' We stand and watch them; it gives me a little breather. After a few minutes, we walk on.

'How're you enjoying it here?' I ask Patji.

'The quality of life, especially for families, is so much better than in London,' he tells me. 'It's a good place to be with young children. And we're right in nature here. There's no pollution.'

Patji speaks to the children in English; Heidi speaks to them in Finnish. Egil is also picking up Norwegian rapidly at the day-care centre he goes to.

'It's really got him to speak more,' says Patji. 'He understands English and Finnish but he didn't use either of them much. Now he's starting to use Norwegian because that's the language he needs to get by at day-care.'

I always regretted that Peter didn't speak Herero to Perivi and Isabel but he said he found it strange to talk to them in Herero when we were living in England and America. By the time we went to Namibia, his established language of communication with them was English and it was difficult to change that. They know a little Herero but not enough to converse, like me.

That evening at their flat, Isabel lounges in front of the television in a low chair. Egil and Meri come and jump on her, squealing with delight as she tickles them and gets up to chase them into their bedroom.

Two days later, we travel further south on another bus, to visit Bente and Uazuvara in Arendal. It's an old port and former capital of Norway. Bente collects us from the bus station in their car and drives us home; Uazuvara hasn't driven since his accident. Their house is on a steep hill. The first floor sitting room has walls that are mostly glass, and overlook the point where the garden drops away and the trees rise up.

Isabel goes to Ida's room. She is one year older than Ida, and they have known each other since they went to pre-school together in Windhoek. Nora joins them. Bente, Uazuvara, Peter and I have coffee in the sitting room. I look out at the trees.

'What a wonderful house.' I say to Bente. 'I feel as if I'm perched in the treetops.'

'It is wonderful,' she says. 'I love it. This is the house we've always lived in, apart from when we were in Namibia. It belonged originally to my mother's aunt.' She pauses.

'But when we moved in, before we were married,' Bente goes on, 'my mother said: "I don't know what your aunt would think." She also found it difficult herself. But I told her she would get used to it. And she did.'

Uazuvara joins the conversation.

'Bente's mother told me: "You've already been married. You're so much older than Bente. You have children and you have no country. I'm not happy about these things."

"Is there anything that I can do to change these things?" I asked her. 'I'll change what I can," I said.'

The following year, he and Bente married.

'Now, 15 years later, our marriage is held up as an example in the family!' Bente tells us, laughing. 'My brothers haven't been so lucky.'

Uazuvara gets up. 'I'm going to the kitchen to make dinner,' he says. 'Come and talk to me.'

We follow, and sit at the small pine kitchen table. He makes us tea.

'Let me tell you what Uncle Stephanus, the head of the family in Namibia, said about Bente,' Uazuvara says.

'What?' I ask.

'He paid Bente the highest compliment. "You have not married a white woman," he said to me. "You have married a human being."' He repeats the original Herero phrase to Peter.

'Kokupire omundu omuvapa, uakupa omundu.'

'Very good,' says Peter, nodding. 'That reminds me of what Inaa said about Jane. She told me that with all my time out of the country, my decision about who to choose as my partner was better than any advice they could have given me. She and Gerson accepted Jane straight away. Inaa said to me, "You are well-suited. This is someone who's been with you and who's stood the test of time."'

The next day, Bente and Uazuvara take us down to the harbour. Little islands with wooden churches and houses surround it. There's a boat festival on. We walk round, looking at yachts, motor boats and little sailing boats. The sun is shining but the wind is cold and I hold my jacket closed around my neck.

'Which boat would you choose, if you could?' Bente asks me.

'A small motor boat,' I say. 'I love the water, but sailing is hard work. I did it with a friend when I was a student. I'd prefer to just potter around the islands.'

They drive us to see the largest island, connected to the mainland by a bridge; others are accessible by ferry. The holiday homes referred to by Norwegians as 'huts' are not as small as they look from the harbour side. Some are quite luxurious, perched on hilltops overlooking the sea. One of Bente's brothers, who works in Oslo, owns a hut here. He and his wife are there for the weekend. They invite us in and give us strong coffee and cakes.

Bente and I go to sit outside and look at the view.

'It's lovely to see you in your own environment,' I tell her.

'You know, my family has a long tradition of serving the community in health and municipal services here,' she tells me. 'I never thought about it until recently, but I see now that this is part of my heritage.'

In her past work as a trade union organiser for the teachers' union, her work with the Namibian solidarity organisation and with the Swedish development NGO in Namibia, and her current job as principal of a newly merged primary and secondary school, Bente is following in their tradition.

196

'But I really miss the Friday breakfast group and the support we gave each other,' Bente says.

'So do I.'

'I had that Friday morning slot entered in my diary as "professional development",' she tells me. 'I valued the professional as well as personal advice.'

'I know,' I respond. 'Talking about ways of dealing with work situations, how to manage difficult meetings, or colleagues. It was something special.'

'I could do with it now,' says Bente.

'How's it going?' I ask. There are more lines around her eyes and she looks tired. Her job, trying to bring two very different schools together, is taking its toll.

'There's resistance from some of the teachers who don't want change,' she tells me. 'But we're getting there slowly. I had a difficult discussion with one senior teacher who doesn't support what I'm doing. He told me that I don't have as much teaching experience as him.'

'So what did you say to him?' I ask.

'"Maybe not," I replied, "but I have experience helping to liberate a whole country!"'

'Good reply!' I say. 'Excellent!'

Bente laughs. 'That's just what Sandy would say!'

Back at the house, at the kitchen table once again, I ask Uazuvara how he's doing.

'I miss the pattern of my life in Namibia,' he says. 'And I don't see much of Bente. She's so busy. She cycles across town, up and down the hills to be at school early in the morning. She comes back late and has many evening meetings.' He pauses to get some carrots and potatoes out of the fridge and proceeds to peel and prepare them, ready to be cooked.

'I'm on my own more now,' he continues. 'The girls are also busy at school and with their own activities.'

Ida, now 15, identifies more with Norway. Nora, who has just turned 13, remains pulled by the soil of Namibia, where she was born.

Then comes the time to travel home on leave. Perivi arrives from the USA for his summer vacation and joins us. Mamadou drives Perivi, Isabel and me down crowded motorways to Frankfurt airport, to take Air Namibia's direct flight to Windhoek. Peter will follow us a week later. We check in and go to the departure lounge, looking for familiar faces; we very often know people on the flights home. The sound of Afrikaans, the Namibian accented English, the brown, black and white faces of the crew and passengers already make us feel at home. We grin at each other.

'Heh, man, I'm going home, man' says Perivi, slipping into an exaggerated swagger, a big smile on his face.

The congestion of Europe falls away as we fly, and we land early in the morning in Namibia. We're met on our arrival by a nephew, Uapiona, who drives us through the hills on the way into town, past the agricultural training institute, a small lodge, a few cattle amongst the thorn trees and farmhouses dotted here and there in the distance. It's a complete contrast to the crowded places and limited views of northern Europe.

Our house is let, so we've arranged to rent a small flat at the bottom of the garden of another house, in a suburb of Windhoek called Eros. It's a self-contained two-bedroom flat, down near a riverbed. We drive halfway down towards it from the road but have to park the car there and walk the rest of the way down a narrower path, with our luggage. Fingers of *vygie* push up from the sandy slope beside the drive, with other, smaller round-leaved succulents providing the beginnings of ground cover.

We go into the flat, put our luggage down and look around. It's simply furnished, clean, with its own kitchen and TV. There's milk in the fridge, tea, coffee, bread and cheese, provided by Deedee and Sandy, and a card to welcome us home.

I choose the bedroom with the best view. I can see the hills of Windhoek – small and thorn-bush covered. Behind them rise the higher hills of Ludwigsdorf where we used to live. Then behind those hills again, reddish brown in the distance, are the Auas Mountains south of Windhoek.

It is winter in Namibia: dry bright weather, with blue skies and sunshine. During the day, it's hotter than the European summer we have left behind, but by four in the afternoon the shadows get longer and the temperature starts to drop.

On our first day, Uanaingi comes to see us at the flat. She walks in with a big smile on her face and hugs us. We ask how she, Diana and Utaa are, and proceed to tell her what we've been doing. Perivi phones his friends and they come in the early evening to take him out for a drink. Isabel phones hers and tells me she wants to overnight with one of them. I phone Deedee and Sandy and we agree to meet at a wine bar. I'm borrowing a friend's car and on my way to the wine bar, I drop Isabel at her friend's house.

I find Deedee and Sandy inside the wine bar; it's too cold to sit outside.

'Yay!' says Sandy, as I walk in. 'Jane is back!' she announces to everyone. 'The Katjavivis are back in town!' I laugh, go up to her and give her a big hug.

'Welcome Jane-Jane!' Deedee says and I turn to hug her too.

'We want to know *everything*,' Sandy says to me as I sit down. I don't know where to start. I just want to bask in the joy of being with these friends again.

Isabel and Perivi stay overnight with their friends so I'm alone in the flat that night. I go to bed but can't sleep because of the cold. It slaps through the windows, penetrating the duvet and blankets. I put on a vest and T-shirt underneath my pyjamas and socks to keep my feet warm. It helps a little, but not enough. There's no heating and no husband to cuddle for warmth. In the end, I fall into a restless sleep, my mind rewinding images of the drive to Frankfurt, the flight, and the faces of my friends.

The birds wake me as the light of dawn arrives and the sound takes me back to so many mornings getting up in the past, getting the children ready for school, and setting off to work. In Brussels, there are almost no birds around our house, despite the trees. The few small ones we do have are chased away by the crows that control our garden territory, except for a lonely green woodpecker that comes sometimes to the lawn.

I have no responsibilities of work here now, no packing and moving to think of, no repairs and renovations to supervise. It's a holiday at home. I allow myself to let go. I breakfast slowly, watching the news. I contact family and friends, relax, watch movies with Perivi and Isabel.

We cook together or go out to eat at favourite cafés, and decide slowly where we want to go and what we want to see.

I drive around the city; going up and down the streets we've lived in, remembering our times there. Our family is rooted in Namibia. The Oxford interlude at the beginning of Perivi's life, and our time in the USA at the beginning of Isabel's, were preludes to this long stretch of life in Windhoek. Every part of the city reminds me of something or someone: events, friends, moments, journeys, and after-school activities when the children were small. Our first house in Pioneers Park where we had a ceremonial planting of a tree in the garden over the placenta that nurtured Bente and Uazuvara's daughter Nora. The veld running alongside the dry riverbed that we walked through to the shops. Then Ludwigsdorf, the drama of seeing that house and falling in love with it, of our move there, and the magnificent view of the mountain. It delights me to see it all again.

Jane, Deedee, Sandy and I go away for the night together that we missed before I left for Brussels. We try a new lodge not far from Windhoek, 15 minutes drive through the mountains, and the same again on a gravel road. The lodge itself is perched on top of a hill, with a view of grassy plains, small thorn trees, a little dam and a waterhole, with the mountains in the distance. I stand outside the reception area and look at the view. It's completely quiet. I feel as though I'm in a temple, on top of the world, in the presence of God in this ancient land.

We stay in two twin-bedded chalets with thatched roofs. Everything is made from local stone; even the walls are covered with local sand rather than paint. There's a spa as well, with an inside pool, a sauna, a crystal bath, and different types of massage, health and beauty treatments on offer. It's the first place like this so close to Windhoek where you can go just for the day and that has such an amazing location. We get a discount, a Namibian 'discovery rate' intended to encourage people to go there, and hope it will last so we can go again for birthday and anniversary celebrations.

We eat dinner in a large thatched dining room, at a table close to an open fire that keeps us warm. The lunches they serve here are self-service buffets but dinner is à la carte. We decide on the game meat – springbok – and order a bottle of red wine to share.

'Unusual for us to be drinking red wine, girls,' I say. 'What's happening to us?' The others laugh. We almost always have white.

While we wait for the food to arrive, I catch up on their news. I ask Sandy about her cancer.

'I've had further incisions and mole extractions and biopsies,' she tells me, pointing to various scars. 'But so far no more malignant cells have been found.'

'Thank God,' I say.

'You know, I've been thinking about it all,' she goes on. She twirls a piece of her hair round a finger in a gesture very characteristic of her. 'I see my cancer as a response to the stress of losing Isobel and nearly losing you.'

I reach out and touch her arm.

'Oh, Sandy,' I say.

'It happens,' she asserts. 'Apparently the cancer rate amongst white farmers in Zimbabwe has shot up since land expropriations began.'

'But the absolute worst,' she says, 'was one test I had to go to Cape Town for.'

'What was it?' I ask.

'A PET scan. It's plutonium based and it's much more sensitive than the MRI scans, so they can really see if there's any cancer anywhere in the body. The doctor here was anxious about one tissue mass, so she sent me down to Cape Town.'

'How do they do the scan?' I ask.

'No, it's the same as an ordinary MRI,' says Sandy. 'You lie down and the bed moves through the tube. But they use radioactive plutonium, and they have to get suited up like they're on the moon or something!'

'Horrible!' says Deedee. 'You've been through a lot, Sandy.'

'We all have,' she says.

Her ongoing medical checks have not stopped Sandy from putting on new productions. Her most recent was 'Animal Farm', with actors from the age of 5 to 18 and three lead actors who are students from Angola.

The meat arrives. We all help ourselves to vegetables from the dishes they bring for us to share.

'You know, when I first came to Namibia,' I tell them, 'I couldn't bring myself to eat springbok. Those cute little animals jumping in the bush. I felt sorry for them.'

'So what changed?' Deedee asks.

'I learnt that springboks are much more eco-friendly because they don't eat all the grass like cattle do, they're browsers not grazers, and the meat is not fatty so it's better for my arteries!'

'Well, bon appétit now,' says Jane. She has told us that she has to return home straight after breakfast the next day because Helao is travelling to Angola.

'So where's Helao going?' Deedee asks.

'He's trying to rediscover his family,' she says. 'You know, Helao was born in Angola, near Ondjiva,' she reminds us, 'although he grew up in Namibia.'

Helao has seen none of these relatives since he was captured by the South Africans in 1966 and imprisoned. He wasn't released until 1984 and after that he went to the UK and studied there until Independence.

'Last year,' Jane tells us, 'his cousins went to a family funeral in Angola and came back telling him that some of his family was still there. It's only possible for him to go now because there is peace in southern Angola.'

'What about landmines?' I ask. Southern Angola has been heavily mined.

Jane raises her eyebrows. 'Yes, well there are still some security issues surrounding their journey, but he wants to go.'

'Helao had 21 other half-brothers and sisters,' Jane warms to her story, 'but was the only child of his mother and father. His father was a rain king and Helao was supposed to succeed him but his mother refused to allow it and removed him from the community. She had converted to Christianity – Catholicism – and didn't want her son to become involved in something she considered heathen. The person who took on that role instead was his favourite sister.'

'Someone should go with Helao with a camera, and film the journey and the reunions,' says Sandy. She immediately starts to phone around to try and organise it. The notice is short, however, and the few filmmakers we have in Namibia are already committed to other projects.

'Helao and other former Robben Island prisoners have been touring schools with a mobile museum in a kombi.' Jane tells us. 'It's mostly an exhibition of photos. They talk to the pupils about their experiences on the Island. They're doing it on a shoestring, with a small budget supported by US funds. A Ministry of Education officer goes with them to help engage the learners, and they end up talking not just about their own experiences but also about the liberation struggle in general. Many of the children haven't been told about the struggle by their parents. It's awful.'

'Do you remember the novel by Kaleni that I published?' I ask them.

'Yes, I read it,' Deedee says.

'It's set in the north of Namibia during the liberation war, when it was at its height,' I remind them. 'South African Defence Force vehicles were trampling people's *mahangu* fields. People were arrested and tortured or killed if they were suspected of supporting SWAPO.' I pause and take a drink of my wine.

'Thank God that's all ended,' Deedee says.

I continue: 'Anyway, one of the lecturers at the University taught this novel to students in the English department. Some of them didn't believe that those things had ever happened. They thought it had all been made up by the author.'

'Memories are short,' says Sandy.

'One generation is all it takes,' I go on. 'It's not yet really in the history books and if you don't tell your children, they won't know.'

A Robben Island Trust has been established to assist the former prisoners. All those who had been on the Island went to the dinner held to launch it, including those from political parties other than SWAPO. Helao was asked to give a talk on their behalf. Jane tells us about it.

'He decided not to talk once again about how hard the conditions had been, about having only one blanket each, about suffering, nor about discovering in the quarries that even a dark black skin does not protect you from being burnt by the sun,' she says. 'Instead he talked about what they had learned and gained from the experience, about learning about themselves, about discovering the good in each other.'

The beds at the lodge are soft and firm at the same time, the duvets light but warm. I don't want to get up in the morning but Deedee and Jane get up early for a walk, and see warthog, springbok and eland – the largest of the antelopes, bigger than a large cow, but still able to jump high fences. After breakfast, we all walk to the waterhole. We see a group of giraffes, including a young one, wandering through the bush to drink, but by the time we get to the waterhole, they have moved on.

When Peter arrives in Windhoek, we go to visit the new bar, El Cubano, that Hugo opened a year after Isobel died. We take our Isabel with us. Perivi is out with friends. The walls are cream-washed with bits of plaster missing in strategic places, giving it an air of slight decay. The overhead pipes are exposed, factory style. Behind the bar, is a map of South America with a portrait of Che Guevara superimposed on it, complete in black beret with red star, a motif reflected in the berets worn by the waiters and the beer mats in khaki cloth, all with the same red star.

Around the top of the walls are framed photographs of revolutionaries (interpreted in a broad sense) chosen by Hugo and his new business partner, who manages the bar. It was opened by the head of the Namibia-Cuba Friendship Society, Minister Andimba Ya Toivo, one of the founders of SWAPO and the most well known Namibian to have been imprisoned on Robben Island. The photos were unveiled at the opening, one by one, with Hugo giving clues as to the identity of each person beforehand. Some are old familiars, others are unexpected. Oscar Wilde is framed by President Robert Mugabe on one side and President Sam Nujoma on the other – neither of them known for their tolerance of homosexuality. Eva Peron is there, as are Osama Bin Laden, Martin Luther King Junior, Gandhi, Malcolm X, Nkrumah, Lenin, Marx, Castro and the South African freedom fighter Joe Slovo (but not his equally revolutionary wife Ruth First, who was assassinated by the South African security forces in the early 1980s). Namibian heroes are also there, including the early twentieth century resistance fighter Hendrik Witbooi, whose portrait graces Namibian bank notes, Ya Toivo himself, and Gwen Lister, an outspoken journalist and editor of *The Namibian* newspaper, which frequently challenges the Government.

Hugo comes over and I give him a big hug.

'What can I get you?' he asks.

Isabel orders a coke and Peter a glass of red wine. Hugo looks at me.

'You know I've created a cocktail named after Isobel – a Tequila Bella,' he tells me. 'It's part tequila, part champagne, with a dash of red bull.'

'Let me try one,' I say. When he brings the drinks, I take a sip of mine.

'Wow, that's strong.' I tell him.

'After two it's hard to get home, they tell me,' he says with a smile.

A quartet of guitar, violin, flute and percussion start up. Hugo, the patron, moves around the room talking to people. He still works as an architect but his life has a different pattern now, with his greater need to be with the children and this new venture into which he has put his heart.

'How are the children coping?' I asked Deedee when we were at the lodge.

'Well, Jan Barend is in his penultimate year at school and seems all right,' she told me. 'He'll soon be off and independent.'

'And Kara?'

'You know what I think,' Deedee said to me. 'I think that Kara has experienced the worst that could ever happen to her and, look, she's survived, so she too will be all right.'

There's a strong support network of friends in Windhoek who hold up Hugo and the children. Some of them tell him not to spend so much time at the bar. The bottom line, I think, though, is that Hugo needs to find a way of living that will enable him to help the children live and grow as well.

As the days turn into August, the wind picks up. The light becomes hazy and you can hardly see the Auas Mountains from the flat. Perivi has to leave to go back to college in the USA, as the new term starts in late August.

Peter, Isabel and I set off to the Waterberg plateau where I first met Deedee. The occasion is a special commemoration at the site of Ohamakari, a terrible battle in the 1904-08 uprising by the Hereros and Namas against German colonial rule. In the aftermath of Ohamakari, colonial forces killed 70 per cent of the Herero and 40 per cent of the Nama people in Namibia. Many died in battle but most died thereafter. The water holes were poisoned and people fled into the Kalahari Desert; a few hundred made it across the desert and settled in Botswana. Concentration camps were established for the survivors. Thousands of Nama prisoners were abandoned on Shark Island off the town of Luderitz on the south coast of Namibia, without food or water. They were simply left to die. In some places, piles of skeletons have been uncovered in the shifting sands, preserved by the dryness of the desert.

There were many colonial atrocities committed in other countries as well, but what marks this out is that there was a written order from the head of the German colonial forces, General von Trotha, stating that all Hereros must leave the land or they would be killed; women and children included. Namibians feel, therefore, that this was genocide.

Now, 100 years after Ohamakari, the affected Namibian communities hold a commemoration of the massacre in a new community centre just outside the nearby town of Okakarara, where Uazuvara comes from. There's a small community hall within a large plot adjacent to where the battle actually took place; hundreds of people gather there beforehand and camp in and around the town.

Herero women wear their long traditional dresses and *otjikaeva*. Women from Okahandja and Okakarara have red dresses with black jackets; the clans from the east, the Ovambanderu, wear green and black; and white for those from the Omaruru area to the west.

Ovahimba also come from the north-west, Kaokoland, where people still live a very traditional life and dress in skins. Herero men are kitted out in uniforms of all types, as they are each year in August when they gather in Okahandja to commemorate their resistance to German colonialism. They march and sing praise songs; some ride horses, throwing up the dust.

Namibians we know who live and work outside the country have returned to be here on this special day. Luther is here too; he proudly wears the uniform of a colonel from the former GDR, which Evelin found for him. People gather to listen to the speeches in a small semi-circular amphitheatre with canvas erected over the platform to give shade to the VIPs. Peter, Isabel and I creep into the back there and manage to find seats. Chiefs from the Herero communities are there, and Nama representatives. Herero Chief Riruako has invited King Kauluma of the Ndonga community in northern Namibia, because the Ndonga people responded to the call to join the uprising against German rule, and Riruako presents the King with two magnificent bulls to express the gratitude of the Herero people.

Several Government Ministers and some diplomats are there as well. President Nujoma is represented by the SWAPO Vice-President, Hifikepunye Pohamba. He is one of Nujoma's oldest colleagues, and is now set to succeed him. When President Nujoma was required to step down after 15 years in office, Pohamba was elected as the SWAPO presidential candidate for the elections due at the end of this year, in November 2004.

The Minister of Economic Cooperation and Development, Heidemarie Wieczorek-Zeul, represents the German Government. Before the commemoration, there were calls from Namibia for Germany to issue an apology for the atrocities but the consistent response was that no apology would be forthcoming. At the commemoration, however, Minister Wieczorek-Zeul gives a powerful speech, accepting that what had happened would today be termed genocide and asking for forgiveness. She uses the words of the Lord's Prayer: 'Forgive us Our Trespasses'. 'This', says the Minister, 'is an apology,' and there is a roar from the crowd – some approving and others wanting more.

After the speeches, the Minister lays a wreath at a memorial to Chief Samuel Maharero. A huge sash is wrapped across the wreath, in the black, red and gold colours of the German flag. It also bears the words 'Forgive us Our Trespasses'. As other Government representatives have had to leave by then, Peter is given the Namibian Government's wreath to lay at the memorial alongside that of the German Minister.

We drive back to Windhoek after the commemoration and go straight to the hospital to visit our old friend, Mosé. He's very weak after a series of chemotherapy treatments for chronic leukaemia. We knock on the door to his private room and open it gingerly. Mosé is lying down in bed but he opens his eyes as we enter the room and gives us a small smile. He tries to sit up to talk to us and we adjust pillows behind his back to help make him comfortable. Peter asks him in OtjiHerero how he is. Then he tells Mosé a little about the Ohamakari commemoration and we leave to let him rest.

I'm used to seeing Mosé in his robes as Speaker of the National Assembly, at public meetings and official functions, or at his home with his family around him. He looks so vulnerable in hospital, somehow old and young at the same time, and I'm reminded that we are all mortal, all vulnerable and frail in the face of illness, no matter what we have done or achieved in life.

Sandy, Jane and Deedee continue with the Friday breakfasts, although the numbers are depleted and the venue varies. Just before I leave to go back to Brussels, we go to Hotel Thule for a special breakfast to celebrate my birthday. It's perched on top of one of Windhoek's hills, at the edge of a cliff. The restaurant has a semicircular window some 15-20 metres wide, with views over the eastern part of the town – residential areas, the shopping centre of Klein Windhoek, schools, the weather centre, and then more hills. The ground drops away immediately beneath. We choose a table where we can look out.

'It's spectacular here,' I say. 'What a wonderful place to have breakfasts. You should come here every week.'

'I was reluctant to come here at all,' Jane tells us. 'It used to be a private house, and I thought it was here that Helao washed windows as a contract worker long ago. But then I discovered that he had worked in some houses nearby, and I felt free to come.'

We are quiet for a moment, remembering how things used to be.

'Come on, let's get something to eat,' I say.

The breakfast is a set-price buffet, with a spread of cereals, fresh fruit, bread, cheese and cold meats, and the option of ordering hot food as well.

'Wow,' says Deedee. 'Look at all this.'

We start with muesli and croissants. A waitress comes to offer tea and coffee; 'Jane's right,' says Deedee. 'We should come here more often.'

'Time to move on,' I suggest to them, and the conversation turns towards transitions.

'Freddie's just turned 13, you know,' says Jane. He's the youngest of all our children.

'Tell us about Freddie's party,' Deedee says.

'Well, it was a sleepover,' Jane explains. 'I had defined it as a 24-hour Boys-to-Men challenge and the boys were rather nervous when they came.'

'How many?' asks Deedee.

'Nine,' says Jane. 'I opened with a discussion about what it means to be a man – what they thought was manly behaviour. And they said the usual things about being tough and strong. Then I asked them to think of the men they admired and to describe what they liked about those men, and the qualities they identified were kind, sensitive, understanding – not the traditional 'masculine' traits.'

She asks the waitress for more tea and continues with her story,

'I organised various activities for them, including go-carting up a mountain outside Windhoek, but first I said they had to choose a name for their group – their age-set – which they could keep and remember and enjoy into the future. I told them they must find a democratic way of deciding on the name. So they discussed it for an hour and then came up with "The Fruit Loops".' She starts to chuckle.

'Fruit Loops?' asks Sandy.

'Yes! Because they're multi-coloured, juicy, and 'just add milk!'

We laugh out loud. People at other tables turn from their quiet conversations to look at us.

'This place is a bit posh for us,' says Sandy.

'Maybe what you mean is that we can't be so loud here,' says Jane and we laugh again.

We go back to the buffet table and order eggs – scrambled for me, fried for Deedee.

'Hard, please,' Deedee tells the chef. 'They must be hard.' She calls across to Sandy who is still sitting at our table.

'Aren't you having anything, Sands?'

'No. Ted made me porridge,' she says.

The chef tells us that the waitress will bring our food to us and we return to the table.

'Thinking about transitions', Sandy says, 'I have to tell you that a wave of confidence has come over me in the past year. For the first time, I really feel I know what I'm doing. I feel that I'm part of a community of women, around the age of 50, who are confident and comfortable with ourselves.'

We wonder if it is hormonal. As the oestrogen winds down in middle-aged women, do we get the equivalent of a little shot of testosterone? How come men always seem to think they know what they are doing from the age of three?

'It's true,' I say. 'Women of our age do have confidence and knowledge and experience, and the years of child-rearing are largely over, except for possible ongoing conflict with teenagers.' I pause. 'Though even teenagers have a pattern that's predictable and regular, if only we could stand back and see it.'

There are other transitions in Sandy's life as well. We had tried to organise for her to come to Brussels earlier in the year, to celebrate her 50th birthday with us, but the plans were overtaken by the death of her mother. She had been ill for years but had a wonderful way of putting it aside, pausing to rest when necessary but living a full life. Many times, Sandy rushed to Zimbabwe to be with her, as they thought her mother was dying; many times, her mother lived on.

'Tell me about your mother,' I say.

'I felt so sad, confused and lonely,' Sandy says. 'My daughter had just left school and was shining, while my mother was fading. They were both leaving, two very important people in my life, on two different journeys. I felt like the bridge between two generations.

'But the time I was in Zimbabwe with my Mom was given to me as a gift,' Sandy continues. 'It was a time to re-assess myself, my family, and my values. I learned how to do all the nursing things I usually leave to my sister. I'm not a natural nurse but I did it and felt good about it. I realised that there is nothing more rewarding and sadder than being needed and being needy all at once.'

I put my hand on her arm. 'It's something to be able to do that, Sandy,' I tell her. 'It's not easy.'

Sandy calls the waitress for more coffee and continues.

'Mom was truly gracious and dignified. She had a grace of giving in her illness. She was beautiful, soft, vulnerable and strong. Dad said a prayer each day before she went to sleep: "Dear God, Be with us in this circle of love," is how he always began. Mom would then sleep and we would go and watch the most gruesome TV murder series we could find!'

When the end finally came, Sandy's mother was cremated but there were fuel shortages in Zimbabwe so the crematoriums couldn't function. They had to go through the Hindu community, and be accepted into it, to be allowed to use their wood-fired cremation facilities. Sandy gathered up her mother's ashes herself and the family scattered them in the bush, not far from where her mother had been born.

Shortly before I'm due to return to Brussels, Deedee calls me to join her for coffee while she's at the hairdresser. We talk while she waits for her hair to be washed.

'Tell me how your work is going,' I say to her.

'Well, you know, I've been doing a lot of work on HIV/AIDS programmes,' she tells me. 'I worked with the Ministry of Health on their strategic medium-term plan.'

'That's crucial work, Deedee,' I say.

'It's a path into the policy-making and implementation process that can affect everyone's lives,' Deedee responds. 'I enjoy it because of that, but I still do a lot of work on early childhood development. People are emphasising the problems of AIDS orphans right now, but I think we shouldn't only focus on the HIV/AIDS aspect but on the wider issue of all vulnerable children.'

The hairdresser calls Deedee to the basin, washes her hair, and escorts her to a chair in front of a mirror. I look around for another chair and pull one up to sit by her.

'The same as usual,' Deedee tells the hairdresser. 'A little bit off but not too short, please.' She looks at me through the mirror.

'You know, I went with Jane to Angola to work on a project there, and we met up with Tricia. She's teaching at the International School outside Luanda.'

'How is she?' I ask

'Well, many of the pupils there are children of expatriate families who've come to Angola to work in the oil industry and they're really cut off from Angolan society,' Deedee says. 'The school itself is in its own separate complex, with accommodation for the staff inside its grounds. Tricia's not particularly happy in that environment.'

She talks about the huge contrasts between the wealthy and the mass of the people in Angola.

'There's great poverty, poor transport, little infrastructure, and a great lack of health resources. It makes me so angry,' she says. 'All that oil wealth, and who benefits from it?'

Then she tells me that it looks as if Tricia will not be returning to Namibia, as her husband Richard has got a job in Zambia after his contract in Namibia came to an end.

'Sad, but we are happy for them,' says Deedee.

'What a shame for Namibia to lose them,' I say. A gentle man, a teacher in all the best senses of that word, Richard has contributed much to Namibia, since long before Independence – training people, building capacity, encouraging their growth. Tricia too, even though she was never really happy with the schools in which she taught.

Then Deedee switches her attention to me.

'But what about you, Jane-Jane? Tell us more about Brussels.'

'Well,' I reply. 'The role of a diplomatic wife is very vague. You can make of it pretty much what you will. Sometimes I feel I'm property manager at the residence.' I pause while the hairdresser asks Deedee to bend forward so she can get at the hair at the nape of her neck.

'Some diplomatic wives say that their job is to eat for their country,' I continue. 'I say that my job is to be charming and elegant, provide good food, and talk about Namibia. Any two of those three at one time, I can do. Trying to do all three together is exhausting!'

'But what do you *want* to do?' Deedee asks.

'I don't know,' I reply. 'I don't know what I'm supposed to be doing. I'm also not sure what to expect of myself. There are still times when I'm overcome by tiredness and have to stop everything and rest, so I don't like to promise anything.'

Do I try to get fit and continue life as normal, glad to have had a narrow escape from my brush with death? Do I make big changes and do things I always wanted to do, before I die? Do I acknowledge that I'm damaged but can function and find some middle path of a changed existence where I can do some things but not quite what I used to do?

There are times when I don't think I should be here at all. I was on my way through the door that Brigitte and Isobel had passed through. Medical intervention stopped me, but I don't know what I'm supposed to be doing now.

'What about your writing?' Deedee asks me.

'Well, I've started another short story, but it's going slowly,' I tell her, and then continue: 'Do you remember the idea I had about doing a series of books for children about the regions of Namibia? So many Namibians don't know what regions other than their own look like. I thought I might explore that idea and see if I could begin to develop something that could be used as additional material in schools.'

I talk about how I would like the books to look and what they might contain. Deedee turns towards me and the hairdresser has to pause.

'Jane, listen to yourself, Deedee says. 'You are beginning to plan.'

As I prepare to return once more to Europe, to move on with my life, I think about these women who have supported me so well. We all had children to look after, and husbands. We all worked but tried to be the sort of mothers who spend time with their children, watch over their homework and school projects, encourage them to do extra-mural activities – music, dance, sport – and take them there in a town without public transport. We all wanted quality time with our husbands, too.

None of us was indigenous to Namibia. We came from outside and perhaps we therefore needed each other more. Our friendships grew over a long period of time and helped create the trust we had in each other.

We were witty and funny and silly and wise and helpful to each other. The Friday breakfasts became something we all looked forward to, each of us taking things there that we needed to share, unravel, explain and pick over. We all offered something to the discussions but dominated them at different times. All of us had our repetitive threads that the rest of us began to recognise so that we could say 'Yes, but you tend to...' All of us knew each other's work and many of the players, since we were living in a small town. All of us accepted the common context of what we were trying to do – nation-building in a new Namibia. It was a rare and special time.

PART 4

Listening to the wind

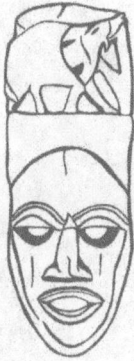

Back in Brussels, I'm no longer the new girl. I now know my way round our diplomatic world and I'm strengthened by our visit home. Isabel sees she has not lost her Namibian core. She stops fighting our move and begins to refer to the house in Brussels as 'home' as well as Namibia – something she had hitherto refused to do. She gets involved with more activities at school and makes more friends.

Perivi moves into a flat in Syracuse, sharing with another student. We talk to him occasionally on the phone, although the time difference makes it difficult to get hold of him. We chat to him online as well, under Isabel's guidance, as this is the first time Peter and I have ventured into this aspect of the internet.

As we turn into 2005, Peter and I start to travel more round Belgium together. We discover mediaeval towns with long histories and long walls, small streets, castle towers, winding rivers, and cobblestones. We visit one such town in the Flemish-speaking region, Mechelen. It's a 30-minute drive from our house and is where Concepcion lives. I've seen the name on road signs and assumed it was a suburb of Brussels. When we get there, however, we discover that in the sixteenth century it was the capital of The Netherlands, with two cathedrals, many former cloisters and lots of bells.

Two teachers from the Royal Academy of Fine Art in Mechelen meet Peter at a dinner and decide to adopt Namibia as the theme for their third-year ceramics class. They come to the embassy to discuss it with Peter and he calls me in to join them. Neither of them has visited Namibia; nor have any of the students. I lend them books of ours and magazines from the embassy, so they have visual information about the country to share with the students.

They plan to hold an exhibition of the final pieces and, a few months later, I visit the college to see how the students' work is progressing. I imagine they will be working on a variety of pots, but there are sculptures, two- and three-dimensional reliefs, animal motifs, abstract renditions of the Herero *otjikaeva* headdress, models of ostrich eggs with textured and painted surfaces, profiles of children's heads, human forms and life-size ceramic warthogs. I'm surprised and impressed by the range of images and ideas, the different ways of working with clay and firing it.

I describe the artworks to Peter when Mamadou takes me back to the embassy.

'They're really beautiful,' I tell him.

'How are the plans for the exhibition working out?' he asks.

'They want your help,' I say, 'regarding time and place.' Then I have an idea: 'Let's get in touch with Joseph Madisia and share this with him.'

Joseph is one of Namibia's foremost artists and I've worked with him in the past when he illustrated some covers and children's books I published. He's now Director of the National Art Gallery in Windhoek.

We send Joseph photos of the students' finished work and ask him to do a foreword for the catalogue of the exhibition. He does so, congratulating the students on the way they've captured the essence of Namibian forms and environment.

'Each nation has its own values and belief systems – their own collective truths,' he writes. 'However, truth is not absolute. It is through appreciating each other's art, material culture and natural environment that we are able to return to our own particular values from a new, refreshed angle.'

The exhibition is held in the cloisters of a former monastery in Mechelen, along a wide corridor that goes round the quadrangle. Peter decides to use the opening as an occasion on which to celebrate Namibia's Independence Day. Five hundred guests from the diplomatic community, the European Union, businessmen and women and other newfound friends, join us. It's the day our new President, Hifikepunye Pohamba, is sworn in. He led SWAPO to another victory in the recent general elections and will be Namibia's second President. We feel proud of this transition of leadership after 15 years of independence, and recognise its importance to the building of democracy in Namibia.

Peter and I and two embassy officials line up to greet the guests as they arrive. Isabel stands with us as well and the guests shake her hand and greet her too. After everyone has gathered, Peter welcomes them. He introduces the exhibition and talks more generally about Namibia.

I walk round, talking to different groups of people. Isabel comes to join me and we look at the artwork together.

'It reminds me how much I enjoyed working with clay at home,' she tells me.

She has shown artistic promise since primary school. I realised it first when her class was set the task of making something out of tin cans for a recycling project. Most of her friends made ashtrays or candle holders.

'What are you going to do?' I asked Isabel at the time.

'I'm going to make a fish,' she replied.

I was sceptical. But she cut two drinks cans into small oval pieces that she used as fish scales, and glued them onto a papier-mâché base she made so that they overlapped each other. She cut longer pieces of tin for the tail and stuck two pop-up plastic bottle tops on the head as eyes. It was a magnificent, multi-coloured fish.

One of our Honorary Consuls invites Peter and me to visit Ghent, another mediaeval Flemish town and a port that dominated European trade from the 12th to the 16th centuries. The Consul is a medical doctor who visits Namibia regularly to hunt, and who has invested in a chain of luxury lodges in Namibia. He arranges for us to meet the Governor of the region and the Mayor of the city.

We have a strict official programme and are told to leave Brussels at eight in the morning, so that we arrive at the outskirts of Ghent at the same time as the traffic police who will escort us into the city. But we leave ten minutes earlier and the police have not yet arrived at the agreed place when we get there. We turn back on the highway and loop round and round the intersections and then try again. This time, a police car and two police motorbikes are waiting for us and they lead us into the centre of the city.

Ghent's skyline is dominated by a belfry tower with 54 bells. Its old quay and canals are lined with tall, thin, gabled buildings, with facades from different centuries and styles. A central church and market square date back to the 1200s. Market day is on Fridays and has been so for over 700 years.

We meet the Governor in a dark, wood-panelled room in one of the city's many historic buildings. We exchange greetings and he and Peter have a short discussion about Ghent and Namibia. The Governor presents Peter with an illustrated book about the history of the area and Charles V, ruler of the Holy Roman Empire in Europe in the sixteenth century, who was born in Ghent. Peter gives him a decorated ostrich egg in a stand. Then we're taken to meet the Mayor and go with him and his wife for lunch on a boat while we tour the harbour. Nowadays, the port handles a wide range of goods: car components, steel, fertilisers, paper, and wood. There are huge container ships, terminals for scrap, recycling and fruit juice, and the industries that have grown up alongside.

I join Peter in discussions with the Mayor and his party about developments in Namibia, possible business links with Ghent, and assistance with our port in Walvis Bay. I enjoy contributing to this side of Peter's representation work.

We go to Ghent again some months later for a ceremony at the university to confer Honorary Doctorate degrees to international figures. We're late for the ceremony because the streets are narrow and one-way, and Mamadou can't find out how to get us to the front door. He succeeds in the end and we slip quietly into the inner chamber of the University Senate, a circular, domed hall with tiered seats, on which sit a bank of academics in their black gowns with stoles of different colours.

Six people receive Honorary Doctorates and an oration is given for each of them in turn, detailing their work and their contribution to world knowledge. Then they go up to receive the degree and give their own speech of acceptance. I'm reminded of Peter's university days and am hit by nostalgia for the whole academic world. I reach for Peter's hand.

'It makes me really miss UNAM,' I whisper to him and he nods in agreement.

The high point of the ceremony is the award of an Honorary Doctorate to Archbishop Desmond Tutu. He's being honoured for his contribution to peace and progress in South Africa, especially his role as Chair of the Truth and Reconciliation Commission in the aftermath of apartheid. The orator says that the Archbishop's whole life has embodied the most serious commitment to equality, justice and love.

'Democracy and freedom are fragile things,' he says, and praises 'the moral code of Desmond Tutu and his great personal engagement'.

Archbishop Tutu, familiar from photos and television images, short and round, with a balding head and little glasses, walks forward to be capped and gowned by the Rector. He is filled with love and a great sense of fun and he starts his acceptance speech with a joke about himself and continues with a joke about God being a black woman. I don't really take in what else he says because I start to weep. I'm overcome by his goodness and by the wonderful reality that apartheid has been defeated. I feel privileged to have been part of the social/political movement that brought about change in Southern Africa.

At the reception that follows in a high-ceilinged university hall, Peter and I push our way towards a table where drinks are being served and help ourselves to glasses of champagne. We reach for canapés from waiters who squeeze through the crowds, circular trays held high over their heads.

Peter finds Archbishop Tutu and congratulates him. They met long ago in London and know each other. Peter introduces me to the Archbishop.

'I'm truly honoured to meet you,' I say but I have no further words to express the depth of what I feel. Others bustle between us and someone sweeps the Archbishop away for a conversation elsewhere.

Isabel and I want to be able to talk to people from the Flemish community and we start a course in Dutch. For three hours each Saturday morning, we attend a class at a nearby language school. Isabel is committed enough to forgo late parties on Friday nights that would render her too tired to go to the class.

I find the written Dutch not too difficult to understand, drawing on some German I learned in school and the Afrikaans I've picked up in Namibia, but speaking Dutch is really difficult for me. The words come out sounding either like German or Afrikaans. Isabel laughs at me as I struggle and I find myself wishing that I had learned Afrikaans properly – I who had always resisted it in the assertion of English as Namibia's new official language since Independence.

I want to continue my French as well, and I undertake another course with Nita, Ana and the others. We start to meet occasionally for lunch at different restaurants across town. A bit slowly at first but then more fluently, we converse in French. We search out restaurants with different types of cuisine – Chinese, Italian, Indonesian, Portuguese. Ana keeps a journal with details of what we eat and what the dishes contain.

As summer comes, Ana, Nita, Naomi, Maki and I venture further afield and go on a day trip to the Belgian coast, to the small seaside town of Knokke. We meet at the Central Station in Brussels. Its interior is old and grimy; the platforms are in dark tunnels that fill with the noise and dust of arriving and departing trains; the train itself is diesel, the carriages quite old but clean. Perivi has just arrived for his summer vacation, and he and Isabel come with us as well. The three of us are planning to continue our journey by train after lunch, to meet up with Peter in Bruges.

When we arrive in Knokke, we walk down from the station through the main street, popping in and out of shops, looking at shoes, handbags and clothes.

'*Ce n'est pas trés interessant pour Perivi* – It's not very interesting for Perivi,' says Ana. But he's in a relaxed mood and doesn't mind trailing after all the women. Nita shows a particular interest in the handbags.

'*Nita, tu as déjà achetais beaucoup de sacs cet ans* – You've already bought a lot of handbags this year,' Ana tells her.

Nita laughs. She turns to look at Ana, her thick black hair swinging across her face as she does so.

'*Mais regarde ce petit sac jaune. C'est mignon* – Look at this cute little yellow bag,' she says, but she doesn't buy it.

The wind is blowing and, as we arrive at the beach, we're hit by the full force of it, strong and cold, coming off the sea. I had wanted to take my shoes off and put my feet in the water, but it's too cold for that.

We look around at different restaurants and choose an Italian one not far from the beach. We sit on the veranda outside, in cane chairs round a wooden table. The wind still gets to us and we keep our jackets on.

'*Je vais prendre de la soupe,*' I say, hoping some soup will warm me up. Ana, Nita, Maki and Naomi go through the menu in detail before deciding what to order. Perivi and Isabel choose pizza.

While we're waiting for the food, Maki's cell phone rings. She answers it and speaks rapidly in Japanese. A look of shock comes across her face and her tone changes. We slow our chatter and watch her. When the call is over, she explains.

'*C'était ma mère* – It's my mother,' she tells us. '*Elle m'a demandait si j'étais en Beligique ou à Londres* – She wanted to know if I was in Belgium or in London.'

'*Mais pourquoi?* – Why?' we ask.

'*Il parâit qu'il y a eu une bombe à Londres* – Apparently there's been a bomb in London,' she explains. '*Quelques cents personnes sont tués* – Hundreds of people have been killed.'

We fall silent and then our questions come. Who? What Where? When? How? The wonders of modern communication mean that we have heard from Japan about something happening only 150 kilometres away from us, across the Channel, but we have no further information and no answers to our questions.

The news casts a sombre mood over us and after we've finished lunch we return straightaway to the station. The others head back to Brussels while Perivi, Isabel and I board a train to Bruges.

We arrive half an hour later, buy a small map at the station, and walk to the hotel where Peter has been staying for a two-day meeting, and where he's booked extra rooms for Perivi and Isabel. We cross a mediaeval square and go down the side of a canal lined with houses that are hundreds of years old. It's pretty, but I don't really pay attention because I'm worried about family and friends in London. As soon as we get to the hotel, I go up to our room and turn on the television, to find

225

out what's happening. It's 7 July 2005 and a series of bomb attacks on underground trains in London, and a bus, have killed 56 people and wounded 700 others. The beauties of Bruges, a thirteenth century port, dubbed the Venice of the North, are overlaid for us with images of death and destruction.

I look in horror at the television images of people emerging from the London Underground stations, confused, injured, covered in dust, and I try not to imagine what it must be like to be in an explosion underground. I pray that no one I know has been hurt, although part of me thinks that means that I hope someone else has been hurt instead. I use the hotel phone and call my parents to see if they've heard from my brother and his children and other relatives in London. They have no news. The cell phone networks in England have been closed for security reasons and they can't get hold of anyone. I try again later and by then they have heard from everyone; all our relatives are safe and well. My parents have also spoken to my sister, Helen, who called them from Mexico when she heard the news. My parents, in their mid-eighties, act as the family information hub.

I discover that Helen's son Daniel narrowly escaped one of the bombs. He's been working in London on a month's internship in the financial sector. Always known for his love of eggs for breakfast, he had no eggs in the flat that day, so he left for work a little early to buy an egg sandwich on the way. He caught a train before the one he usually got, which was one of those that were blown up.

A few days later, it's announced that the suicide bombers responsible for the bombings came from Leeds, where I grew up. Perivi hears from one of his Namibian friends who has been living and working in the same neighbourhood of Leeds that the bombers came from.

'It's all too close,' I say to Peter.

At the end of July, three weeks after the bombings, Perivi, Isabel and I travel by train to England for Rachel's wedding (Sarah's eldest daughter) and Jon, her long-term boyfriend. They've been together for over ten years, since they were teenagers. Peter isn't able to be with us as he's in Windhoek for a meeting of Namibian ambassadors.

When we alight from the Eurostar train at Waterloo station in London, we see armed police carrying submachine guns and wearing bulletproof vests. They patrol the platforms and watch over the entry and exit points where tickets are checked. The week before, London policemen shot and killed an unarmed Brasilian, Jean Charles de Menezes, thinking he was one of the London bombers. He came out of a block of flats they were watching and they chased him onto a tube train and shot him seven times. They didn't check that he was the man they were looking for.

'I'm not wearing a scarf over my hair, you can be sure,' Isabel told me before we set off from Brussels. It's a style she's fond of and looks good in, with the ends of the scarf tied round her hair in a tight knot at the back.

'I'm not carrying my things in a rucksack,' said Perivi. The London bombers carried their bombs in backpacks.

They're both nervous that police and other passengers will be suspicious of them because of their brown skins.

In the hills of Wales, however, where Rachel and Jon's wedding takes place, there are no such anxieties. Their wedding ceremony and reception are held in a seventeenth century house, Treowen, with panelled rooms, wide wooden staircases, large gardens and views over hills and woodlands. It's big enough to accommodate many of the guests overnight as well. A team of family members and other helpers prepare a vegetarian feast for the reception.

'Wait until I get married,' says Perivi to his cousins when he realises there is no meat. 'My wedding reception will be meat-only!'

After the speeches and the meal, Rachel and Jon open the dance-floor. My parents join them, and then the rest of us. The dancing continues through the night while the older generation goes to bed. We wake the next morning to eat more and go on to visit the ruined Raglan Castle and then back to my parents' home.

A fortnight later, we host a weekend gathering in Brussels for the English side of the family. There are 22 of us in total, spread in bedrooms across the residence, with five young men lined up on the floor of the annexe flat that has been cleaned out especially for the purpose. Feasting, talking, playing football on the lawn, Isabel (now 16) leading her cousins round Brussels at night and back on the first tram at dawn.

Most of the diplomatic spouses I encounter are talented, energetic women who have put their own careers on hold to follow their husbands round different diplomatic postings. They promote their countries with little recognition and no pay. Some of them find courses to study in order to have more to their lives. Few have the opportunity to follow their professions while they're posted abroad. But I'm one of the lucky ones, because I've been able to do some consultancy work.

After the review of the women's writers' association, Femrite, in Uganda, I was asked by the same Dutch NGO to jointly facilitate a workshop in late 2004 in Nairobi, for writers' associations they support in Uganda, Tanzania, Zimbabwe and Kenya. The aim of the workshop was to share experiences and ideas in the promotion of writing and reading in the respective countries. There was a strong focus on women writers and one of my inputs was to present a section from my report on Femrite in Uganda. I also gave a short paper on 'Developing Women Writers'.

Ruth, a Kenyan publishing consultant and book activist who runs the East African Book Development Council, was the other facilitator, and since she was local, she had the more onerous task of the practical organisation of the workshop. We emailed each other in advance regarding the objectives of the workshop, its structure and programme. When the time came, I flew in through Amsterdam for four days, presented my papers, joined in the discussions and chaired some of the sessions.

'Too often, in too many countries, women are silenced when they try to speak out about their lives, about their relationships, about the laws they are subject to, about their ambitions and about their sexuality,' I wrote in my paper. 'Women who speak out and who write out are often labelled "unfeminine" and "unAfrican".'

I recalled the strong tradition of African women writers, nevertheless and the increase since the late 1990s in the numbers of women who have been published.

A surprise visit from Kenyan novelist Ngugi wa Thiong'o and his publisher Henry Chakava, arranged by Ruth, was an unexpected and delightful extra. Ngugi talked about his writing and the political repression he experienced. Henry spoke about the interference of government officials when he published Ngugi's work, and their attempts to block the publications. I had worked with Henry in the past in the African Publishers' Network (APNET), as he is one of the founder members.

I stayed at the Nairobi Safari Club, where the conference was also held, a high-rise hotel that didn't really live up to its name. Each morning, I was woken by the muezzin calling the faithful to prayer. The mosque was not close to the hotel and the sound was muffled by the other noises of the city, the walls and windows of the hotel and the curtains in my room. But I looked forward to hearing it in the morning and at the end of the day.

Now, in mid 2005, I join Ruth and another consultant in a mid-term review for donors of the African Books Collective (ABC). ABC was set up in the late 1980s by a group of African publishers to market and distribute their books outside Africa, and has a secretariat in Oxford, in the UK. Partially funded by donors and partially generating its own income from sales, the ABC has done much to promote African books and African publishing. They represented New Namibia Books, and the income from international sales helped to make it possible for us to publish further general titles. Their work has benefitted other independent publishers across Africa in similar ways. Over 100 African publishers are now members.

I join Ruth and Nigel, the lead consultant, in Oxford for interviews with Mary, the Director of ABC, and its staff. We design a questionnaire that's sent round African publishers who are members of the Collective and interview partners in the UK and internationally. My particular focus is on the commercial realities confronting African publishers, the role of ABC in their activities, and ways to build up ABC sales.

The ABC office and warehouse are located in the west of Oxford, near the publishing office where I first worked as a book editor, and the river and canal along which I used to walk to work nearly 25 years ago. It's strange to be in Oxford again after having lived there long ago. Because it's such an old city, much of it looks exactly the same, but Peter's and my lives have changed a lot since we lived there.

'I love Oxford,' I tell Mary. 'It's a beautiful city and it holds many good memories. But normally I don't like to go back to places where I've lived or worked. I like to go forward.'

There are still many people I know in Oxford but I don't have the time to contact them. Nevertheless, I walk down St Giles towards

Brown's cafe where Peter and I used to often meet friends for coffee or a meal, and think it would be perfectly possible to meet someone I know. As I do so, I sense rather than see someone coming up behind me and I turn. It's Dwight, an old friend who we knew well when we were in Oxford, and who was at our wedding, but whom I haven't seen for ten years, since his own wedding in Oxford in the mid 1990s.

'What? Jane!' he exclaims. He's astonished to see me. 'What are you doing here? Is Peter with you? How are you?'

He looks very much the same, tall and thin, with a slight Afro hairstyle and a freckled face. His American accent is still there. We give each other a kiss on the cheeks and stop to catch up briefly with each other's news.

'I'm sorry, Dwight, but I have a meeting and don't have much time. It seems awful to run off quickly after not seeing you for so many years, but I have to go. Come and see us in Brussels,' I say.

We exchange contact details and he promises to visit us.

How far we've come, I think, since we were in Oxford. How far Peter has come, from postgraduate student to ambassador; how far Namibia has come, from the liberation struggle to a new democracy; and me, from a newly married book editor to publisher, book activist and mother of young adults. Much of what we dreamed of then has come to pass.

I return to Brussels to write my part of the report and am glad that I'm not solely responsible for the whole evaluation, as I was in Uganda. I submit sections I'm working on to Ruth and Nigel. We merge it with the parts they're working on and get comments on the draft from ABC and the donors for whom we're doing the evaluation.

One of the tasks we've been given is to comment on how the work of ABC helps in poverty reduction – the new focus of donor agencies. We emphasise how ABC produces a variety of different outputs and outcomes – for authors, publishers, readers in countries of the global North, the spread of ideas, a contribution to employment creation within Africa, and African economic, educational and cultural development.

We have to go to Oxford at the end of the year to present the report to a full meeting of ABC and the donors. The meeting is held in a side room of the Randolph Hotel in the centre of Oxford. I stay with my parents and drive up to Oxford for the day. As I walk into the room, I look at everyone seated round the table and go round to greet them. The members of the ABC Council of Management are colleagues with whom I've worked in APNET in the past, and who've encouraged my own publishing ventures and those of others: the chairman, Walter Bgoya, a well-known publisher from Tanzania; Henry, from Kenya; Akoss, a publisher of illustrated children's books from Ghana; and Dayo from Nigeria. Apart from Henry, I last saw them at Victor's funeral in 2002.

I go back to Brussels to prepare for Christmas. Perivi returns for two weeks with everything sorted out for a transfer to a college in Los Angeles, where he will start in the New Year, January 2006. He has always been interested in practical film production and has found a course that offers just that.

Two of Isabel's friends come from Namibia to be with her and she takes them round Brussels and to the snow and ice festival at Bruges, where hundreds of thousands of kilos of ice and tons of snow are shipped in for ice sculptors to work on.

'What was it like?' I ask them when they return.

'It was cold!' says Pendu and Veno laughs in agreement. The temperature inside the hall was well below freezing and they've just come from the hottest season in Namibia.

We are drawn into a sequence of end-of-year parties thrown by different diplomatic friends. A New Year's Eve party for diplomats from countries of the Southern African Development Community (SADC) is hosted by one of our Namibian colleagues from our embassy, and his wife. They have five children and an open, welcoming home. Their eldest daughter Monica is Isabel's age and has become a friend of hers. Isabel loves to visit her at weekends, and stay in their household, which is much livelier than our quiet one.

We spend New Year's Eve dancing. I'm inducted by my southern African sisters into doing the electric slide. Fifteen or more women dance in a group together. We step forward and to the side, backwards and to the side. We bend our right knees up, spin on our left feet and turn to face a different direction, and continue with the original steps, spin and turn again. Laughing, diplomatic distinctions gone, older and younger women dancing together. The men stand round the room, enjoying the spectacle and encouraging us to continue.

Peter and I have become friendly with diplomats from SADC and the Africa, Caribbean and Pacific group of countries with whom he works so much, and whose spouses I meet regularly.

'Have you noticed,' I ask Peter after a dinner with some of these friends, 'that you get on well with the husbands of the women I get on well with?'

'Yes, it's true,' he says.

'But we became friends separately,' I add, 'me with the women and you with the men, not as couples. It's interesting.'

'Some people are much more active and involved than others,' he says. 'And maybe we both like that.'

I decide to become more active and involved in the ACP spouses group. The wife of the Ambassador of Barbados, Cecile, is the Dean – the head – of this group. She draws me in to be co-chair of the organising committee for a gala fund-raising dinner. Yasmine, the wife of the Ambassador of Egypt, is the other co-chair. The other committee members are the wives of the Ambassadors of Suriname, Moenisha; the Eastern Caribbean States, Celia; the Democratic Republic of Congo, Peggy; Niger, Rekia; Malawi, Kelly; and Cecile herself.

The aim of the group's fund-raising activities is to support projects in ACP countries in situations of extreme need. The year I arrived, the group held a gala dinner that raised €20,000 for a children's home in Botswana that caters mainly for AIDS orphans. Last year a similar dinner raised €15,000 for a Mobile Caregivers Programme in Grenada after 80 per cent of the island's infrastructure, and more than 90 per cent of homes, were damaged by a hurricane. The project helps young children from disadvantaged homes in rural areas who do not have access to early childhood education. The Mobile Caregivers' office base and materials were all destroyed by the hurricane.

This year, the gala will be held in aid of communities in Niger and Malawi, where changing climate patterns, droughts, floods, locust infestations and the dependency on rains for crop production have created severe food crises. Two trusted projects – one in each country – have been identified that provide education, medical care, and nutrition for those most in need, as well as support to the surrounding communities through sustainable agriculture and livestock projects. We are aware of the contradictions inherent in planning a dinner to raise funds for people who don't have enough food, but it has proved a successful event in the past, so we carry on.

The gala organising committee meets weekly, in the house of one or another of the members, and we talk for hours. We're all used to organising our own events and have our own ideas of what to do and how to do it, so we discuss every last detail until consensus is reached. We chase around Brussels to printers, draft letters in English or French for embassies and companies from whom we are seeking sponsorship, and hand them over to someone else to be translated so that they are available in both languages. We go to companies, shops, restaurants and hotels, looking for sponsorship and gifts to be drawn as prizes or sold by silent auction. We go to hotels and discuss room size, stages, sound equipment and dance floors. We plan table layouts and try out dishes over lunch so that we can decide on the menu. We sell tickets to the gala and tickets for the tombola.

'It's taking over your life,' says Peter to me one day as I ask yet again for Mamadou's help to drive me to my meetings.

I smile at him. 'Yes, it is rather,' I concede. 'And we don't make decisions the most efficient or simplest way. But it's a wonderful collection of women. I value the friendship that's growing through our work together.'

In the midst of all this, Sandy delights us with a visit, on her way back to Namibia after a reunion in the UK with her father, her sister (who is now settled there) and brother, who has worked in London for some years. I put Sandy in the Jacaranda room and she throws open the window to let in the fresh air. It's April and the central heating is still on to combat the damp cold outside.

'I can't stand being closed in,' she says.

Her energy fills the house. Her enthusiasm fills my heart. We go round Brussels, to Grand Place and the tourist centres, to art exhibitions and museums: a packed three days that take me to places I haven't yet visited in the time I've been in Brussels. We take her to the Music Village, a small, smoky jazz club we've discovered, just off Grand Place, where the music is too loud to be able to talk.

'I want you to meet Nita,' I tell Sandy. 'She's one of the women I've met here, while learning French. She reminds me of Deedee – petite, active, sporty, and full of laughter. I think you'd get on well.'

'I'd like to meet your new friends,' says Sandy.

'Well, I don't know Nita as well as I'd like to,' I say. 'We're usually in a group together with others, talking in French, and it's limiting because my French isn't good enough to have the sort of discussion we would have in Windhoek. But I like Nita and I want to get to know her better.'

I take Sandy to meet Nita at her flat. It overlooks one of the Brussels parks and has an eclectic mixture of decorations: modern surrealist art that her husband Aachim likes, Indonesian masks, photos from both sides of the family on the mantelshelf, low coffee tables and a collection of elephants carved out of different materials – wood, stone, brass and more.

Nita welcomes Sandy in French and breaks into English in order to communicate with her. Her voice sounds quite different from when she's speaking French and I'm surprised to discover she has an American accent. She makes us coffee and Aachim takes a photograph of us together, before Sandy and I move on to visit the museum of musical instruments. They provide headphones that pick up the sound of each instrument as we pass by the display cases from different parts of the world. It's as if the music exists in its own dimension, and by moving in the right direction we can discover it.

After three days, Sandy leaves to go back to Namibia, and I concentrate once again on preparations for the Gala. On the day itself, in early May, the committee members meet at the Sheraton Hotel in the centre of Brussels, where the Gala is being held, and we spend most of the day there. We check on how things have been laid out, set out tables for the silent auction of crafts from ACP countries, and put up information about the projects we are supporting. The tickets are sold out and 300 guests gather that evening at tables of ten – businessmen and women, diplomats, government officials, friends and relatives of the ACP ambassadors and their spouses. The men wear dinner jackets or dark suits; the women, evening dresses or traditional dress – long, flowing and colourful – from different countries around the world. Isabel helps at the tombola, looking grown up and stunning in a little black dress.

We start at 7 p.m. with cocktails, and go on to a three-course dinner. The main course, decided on after much discussion about different food preferences and taboos, is lamb. A Mauritian dance group entertains us between courses and a Caribbean band plays music we can all dance to after we've eaten.

My sister Sarah and her husband Dennis come over from the UK to be with us at the dinner. Luther's partner Evelin joins us from Bochum, and also Gisela, the mother of Luther's daughter Miriam, and her husband Erich, who come from Berlin. The evening is a great success and we raise €30,000.

The Gala is, however, overshadowed by the death of our dear friend Mosé, from leukaemia, and Peter and Luther are not able to be with us because they have travelled home for the funeral. Uazuvara goes as well.

Mosé's death shatters us. Peter has lost one of his closest friends; Isabel is inconsolable at the loss of one of her dearest uncles and I cannot imagine Mosé not being in our lives anymore.

Mosé, Peter, Luther and Uazuvara were like brothers. Mosé grew up in Ovitoto with Luther and Peter. His father and Peter's Aunt Maria, who brought Peter up, were active elders in the church and used to sing together. Mosé's father would talk long into the night with Luther's father about the political situation. Mosé went with Peter and Uazuvara to the Augustineum School in Okahandja, which brought together people from different communities who later became the leaders of Namibia.

All four were from the Herero community and joined SWAPO at a time when it was predominantly an Ovambo organisation. Luther and Mosé even went into exile together across the Kalahari Desert in 1964. They all worked together in exile, developing even stronger bonds of friendship and comradeship, representing SWAPO at offices in different countries. Mosé worked at the United Nations Institute for Namibia in Lusaka, training young Namibians to be ready as administrators once independence came.

Mosé played an active part in SWAPO's election campaign in 1989. He was elected to the Constituent Assembly and contributed to the writing of the Constitution. He was chosen as the first Speaker of the new National Assembly and served in that post for 15 years. He built the new parliamentary system, making it a transparent and effective forum for legislation and debate on national and regional issues. He was instrumental in developing a regional body – the SADC Parliamentary Forum. He was highly respected at home and internationally for spearheading and symbolising Namibia's developing democratic culture.

In 2004, however, Mosé clashed with President Nujoma in the run-up to the choice of Nujoma's successor. While the President came out in support of Pohamba, Mosé nominated the Foreign Minister Hidipo Hamutenya. Nujoma was angry – he had been hoping for a unanimous endorsement of his candidate of choice – and he subsequently fired

Hamutenya. When President Pohamba took office a few months later, a new Speaker was appointed.

Now, in his death, Mosé is recognised as a national hero and is given a state funeral, the very day of our Gala in Brussels. Through the night before, his body lies at his home in the village of Okomakuara, the family sitting with him. At dawn, they drive to Windhoek. The funeral starts in the gardens in front of the National Assembly buildings, in the shade of the Jacaranda trees – the most beautiful green space in Windhoek, and the only space with enough natural shade to protect hundreds of people seated. Because of this, and because of its location, it's often used for state occasions. A eulogy is given by Kerii, his 28-year-old son, whom I have watched grow up. Peter is one of the pallbearers and also speaks. Tributes pour in from the region and around the world, emphasising Mosé as a visionary of great integrity, endowed also with the practical skills of management. The cortege then proceeds to Heroes' Acre, where Mosé is buried.

In his speech, Peter speaks of his and Mosé's 'political baptism' in the hills, mountains and rivers of Ovitoto and the surrounding areas.

'Mosé was one of those young men who joined SWAPO in the early 1960s, along with Uazuvara Katjivena, Luther Zaire, myself and others. The steps taken by those young men contributed significantly, at that time, to the development and growth of SWAPO, giving it a national outlook... During these years we worked together in the party as comrades. For some of this time I was based in London but when I returned to Lusaka I was based at Mosé and Sandra's house. Their home was my home in Lusaka. So it was for many, many Namibians who found warmth and shelter in the Tjitendero family...

'Mosé discharged his duties with absolute dignity and did so much to build a parliamentary regional and international community. Since the sad news of his untimely death was made known, friends and colleagues at home and abroad have spoken about the terrible loss Namibia and the Southern African region have suffered...

'Mosé was a close friend, a comrade and a brother. He was also an extraordinary personality who always had time for everyone, big or small... We will always remember Mosé for his contribution to Namibia's freedom and its subsequent development. We will also carry with us his humanity, his gentleness and openness. These are his permanent gifts to us.'

In the media coverage, Mosé and Sandra are reported as having eleven children – their own biological children and all the other children they look after. I have always been impressed by their capacity to open their hearts and their home to so many, especially young women who needed encouragement and support.

Our daughter Uanaingi joined other women of the extended family, going to the Tjitendero home after Mosé died, to help look after all the people who came to pay their respects. But she cannot be there for the funeral, as her 23-year-old daughter Diana gives birth to her first-born – a son – the day that Mosé is buried. They name him Penaani; it was Mosé's middle name.

After coming to Brussels, my health has improved and I've grown stronger. My pacemaker has kept me balanced, and the medication has controlled the extra heartbeats, disciplining my heart. I continue to have difficulty climbing hills and get tired more quickly than I used to, and if I catch a cold, I feel exhausted; but I've discovered that if I rest and sleep, I usually rise again refreshed.

While organising the Gala, however, I was troubled by recurrent symptoms of discomfort – a feeling of nausea in my throat, a dull ache on my right side, a feeling of obstruction when I bent over to put on tights or socks, and greater difficulty walking because of a feeling of pressure in my chest. I went to the doctor and he did various tests for stomach and digestive problems but found nothing. I cut out meat, wine, anything fatty, raw vegetables, and lived for a few weeks on bread and soup but things didn't improve.

The doctor suggested I might have intolerance to wheat, in which case living on bread was not a good idea, but nothing was found in the relevant tests. He sent me for a CT scan of the liver and, again, everything was clear. The symptoms have continued, however, and I go to see the doctor again.

'I'm slowing down,' I tell him. 'And I'm starting to think it has something to do with my heart,'

'No, no,' he says to me. He's Flemish-speaking but his English is near-perfect, as are his French and German. 'I'm not sure what the problem is but we'll get to the bottom of it.'

After another two weeks and no improvement, I make an appointment directly with the cardiologist and explain my symptoms to him. He does a sonar of my heart.

'Your heart function is further reduced,' he tells me straight away. Apparently my body has been struggling to compensate for what the heart is not doing so well, and this has led to the other problems.

Because it's confirmation of what I suspected, I feel strangely pleased with the diagnosis and don't properly take in its implications.

'The strain on your heart is caused by the irregular heartbeat and I want to start you on some new medicine to control that better,' says the cardiologist. 'It's a good medicine. It'll support your heart more but it can have some side-effects on the liver and on the eyes, and we have to build up slowly to the full dose.' He pauses. 'I'm also putting you on a diuretic that will reduce the fluid you're beginning to retain. That should help you feel better quickly.'

The diuretic makes me lose four kilos in a week and relieves the aches in my liver area, the difficulties I had bending down and the pressure in my chest.

I stay quietly at home, reading and resting. However, the new medication I've been given pushes down my blood pressure, so although the other symptoms have gone, there are times during the day when I feel overwhelmed with tiredness and must lie down.

One day, as Peter and I talk after lunch about his work, I feel suddenly sick and dizzy. My arms tingle and my hands go numb. It's unlike anything I've felt before.

'I feel really weird,' I say to Peter. 'I have to go and lie down.'

He follows me up to our bedroom and I lie down. He sits by me on the bed, picks up my hand and holds it. After a few minutes, he asks me if I'm feeling any better.

'No,' I say. 'Lying down doesn't seem to help.'

'Do you want me to phone the doctor?' he asks but I don't feel like doing anything.

The episode passes after ten minutes and I call the cardiologist, and make an appointment to see him the next afternoon.

The following day, I have a lunch with the International Ambassadrices' Group, the last one of the diplomatic season before the summer holiday. Peter suggests that I don't go but I want to wish everyone a good holiday.

'Besides, you know how it is,' I say. 'Some of them won't be coming back after the summer.' It's the traditional time when diplomatic postings change.

Although I feel quite tired, Mamadou drives me to the lunch. A sudden downpour floods the roads and pavements as we arrive and he jumps out to hurry round to my door with an umbrella to cover me. Nevertheless, my cream coloured shoes and my feet get soaked as I bolt from the car to the door of the host's residence – a large apartment in Brussels' oldest Art Decor apartment bloc that dates back to the 1920s.

Mamadou collects me again after the lunch to take me on to the cardiologist. I describe the episode of the previous day to him.

'I thought maybe my blood pressure was very low,' I say.

'I don't think low blood pressure is the cause,' he replies. 'I'm worried that it might be tachycardia – runs of very rapid heartbeats.' He pauses. 'I want to monitor your heart for a few days to see if there's evidence of this. It can be very dangerous.'

My heart jumps at what he says. Is this the beginning of the deterioration I've feared ever since my heart collapsed three years ago, I wonder? Will this overshadow Isabel's last school year? Will I live to see her establish herself independently?

The cardiologist says he will contact me regarding dates and I go home. We pick up Peter from the embassy on the way.

'How did it go?' he asks me.

'I'll tell you at home,' I say, not wanting to discuss it in the car in front of Mamadou.

When we get to the residence, we go into the kitchen and make ourselves a cup of tea. We can hear the sound of music from Isabel's room upstairs.

'I have to have more tests,' I say to Peter, and I explain what the cardiologist told me. I try to keep my tone light. He looks worried but doesn't voice his fears, and I don't voice mine.

In the week of important public exams for Isabel, at the end of her penultimate year at school, I go into hospital for observation and tests. I try to keep it from her for as long as possible, telling her that I'm going in for a blood test early on the Friday, which is true as that will be the first test, but I don't tell her that I will stay in for other tests as well. I intend to tell her more when she's finished the exams she has to take that day. I've told my parents, however, and they phone to wish me well, after I've already left for the hospital. Isabel takes the call and finds out what is happening. She calls me on my cell phone while I wait in the hospital, an hour before her first exam.

'What's going on, Mummy?' she asks. 'Where are you? What's happening? Grandad phoned and told me you're going to hospital.'

'I'm really sorry, sweetheart,' I say. 'I didn't want to worry you. They want to check my heartbeat over a couple of days so I've come in to do that. I wanted to tell you after your exam, so you wouldn't worry.'

'How could you do that?' she asks, her voice tight.

'I'm so sorry.' I apologise again and wish her all the best in her exam.

The hospital is in the middle of Brussels, near the central shopping area, and opposite the Sheraton where our Gala was held. It's an old building, renovated inside maybe 20 years ago, not new and shiny like the private ones in Namibia or South Africa, but clean and efficient, and the nurses are friendly. All the doctors I encounter speak perfect English, but I speak to the nurses in French.

I have a small private room and the doctors hook me up to a portable heart monitor for a four-day ECG. I can move around but have nowhere really to go, so I sit or lie on the bed most of the time, and reflect. There's a sense of bustle in the corridors outside at times but it's blissfully quiet in my room. My stay turns into a retreat, a time of spiritual renewal.

Three days before I was due to go into hospital, I had received a phone call from Celia, a friend from the gala committee. She's a committed Christian, outspoken in her declarations of faith, answering her phone with the assertion 'Jesus is Lord'. She wanted our meetings to be opened with a Christian prayer, even though there were people of other faiths on the committee, and most of us thought it was therefore not appropriate. We didn't tell Celia what we thought, but tried to avoid her praying by getting started with the agenda very quickly.

'I need to see you Jane,' Celia said to me when she called. 'Can we meet?'

'Certainly,' I replied, feeling intuitively that she was coming to testify about her faith.

We arranged to meet near a little café not far from our house and I waited for Celia outside, but when she came, she didn't want to go in. She asked me to come with her to her car and we got in and sat in the front seats. She looked awkward behind the steering wheel, turning towards me to talk.

'Will you pray with me Jane?' she asked.

'Yes,' I said, wondering what was coming.

Celia hesitated and then spoke.

'A prophetess came to our church last Sunday,' she started. 'She told me that I should go to someone I know who has heart problems, and help to heal them, so I thought of you.'

I was touched by her concern and surprised she knew about my heart. I had told Cecile I wasn't feeling well, that I had a heart condition and needed to rest, but I hadn't given her any more details and hadn't told Celia or the other ACP spouses. I didn't want to draw attention to myself or explain my medical history to everyone.

Celia talked to me about her faith. She prayed for me, asking for me to be healed. She gave me a list of Bible readings and Psalms to read, and her Bible as well.

'I've highlighted a lot of passages that speak to me and give me strength,' she said, 'and I can always get another one.'

'Thank you Celia,' I said. 'Thank you for your care. I really appreciate it. I have a Bible but I haven't read it for a very long time.'

When I packed my bag to come to the hospital, I put my Bible and Celia's list in it, but no other books or reading matter – most unusual for me.

In the quiet of my hospital room, I read the Gospels for the first time in 20 years, and reflect on them. I'm struck by how full they are of stories of healing. I read the Psalms Celia referred me to, and others, and I start to pray. I pray for protection.

> *God is our shelter and our refuge,*
> *A timely help in trouble,*
> *So we are not afraid when the earth heaves*
> *And the mountains are hurled into the sea.*
> Psalm 46

I pray for healing. I want to believe that the power of God can be channelled to perform miracles. I hold onto specific references to the heart in my need to strengthen my own:

> *Truly my heart waits silently for God,*
> *From whom comes my deliverance,'*
> read the words of Psalm 62.
> *In truth, God is my rock,*
> *My tower of strength, so that I stand unshaken.*

Most of the time I'm in hospital, the monitor shows that my heartbeat is irregular but not dangerously so, but on the last day the cardiologist sees evidence of the tachycardia he was looking for. I don't really understand the implications of it, but he tells me that the runs of rapid heartbeat are dangerous and arranges for me to see him at his rooms the next day.

Peter comes with me to the appointment and we go into the cardiologist's room together. We sit on straight-backed chairs side by side, facing the cardiologist across his desk.

'You'll need a different type of pacemaker,' the cardiologist tells me, 'to guarantee you a safer future for the next ten years. I recommend you get a dual-chamber pacemaker with a built-in defibrillator.'

'What's that?' I ask.

'The dual-chamber pacemaker gives a better balance to the two parts of your heartbeat,' he says. 'And the defibrillator can control the tachycardia,' he pauses. 'It's automatic and it gives little shocks to the heart if there's an episode of tachycardia, to stop the rapid heartbeats. It's very effective.'

The thought of something shocking my heart horrifies me and I look in alarm at Peter; he picks up my hand and strokes it. We ask for more information and the cardiologist suggests we think about it and get back to him in a few days' time to arrange an appointment for me to have the new pacemaker fitted. We leave his office in silence, get into the car and Mamadou drives us home. When we arrive, Peter makes us both a cup of tea and I go to his study and do an internet search on the defibrillator. I find more information about it on the website of the American Heart Foundation.

'Apparently, it can also give you a strong electric shock in the case of cardiac arrest,' I tell Peter. I'm stunned by the mere thought of it.

In the Frankenstein stories, electricity is used to kick-start life. It's used by my current pacemaker to make my heart beat. It's used in the pacemaker they're proposing I get, which would shock my heart into a normal rhythm if necessary. Electricity is used to restart hearts and rescue lives but I'm horrified at the idea of this new pacemaker and don't want to have one. However, people who experience spiritual or divine healing talk about a surge of electrical/heat energy passing through them at the moment of healing. Is God like electricity, I wonder – giving light, burning bright, a burning, fearful, awesome force that can create and destroy?

Over the next few days, I sit at home and wonder what to do. Peter is attentive and comes home early from the office to be with me, but I feel frightened and sorry for myself. I know I need to let go of my fear but I can't. Then Celia calls me on my cell phone, saying she felt the need to call me.

'I'm struggling,' I tell her when she asks me how I am.

'Read Psalm 91,' she says, but I don't.

The next day, when Juliet arrives in the morning, she comes into the breakfast room where I'm having coffee. Peter has already left for the embassy.

'I have a present for you, Madame,' Juliet says, and she gives me a cloth with the words of Psalm 91 printed on it.

'Thank you, Juliet,' I say. 'That's very kind of you,' and I glance through it.

Later that day, Sandy phones from Namibia to see how I am.

'I'm having a hard time,' I say.

'I know, my love, I know,' she responds. 'I just felt I needed to call you. You know, my Dad always turns to Psalm 91 when he's down. You should read it.'

These three separate references to the same Psalm bring me much comfort, as do the words of the Psalm itself when I finally read it:

> *Whoever goes to God for safety,*
> *Whoever remains under the protection of the Almighty,*
> *Can say, 'You are my defender and protector, you are my God,*
> *in you I trust.'*
> *You will keep us safe from all hidden dangers and from all deadly*
> *diseases. Your faithfulness will protect and defend us,*
> *We will be safe in your care.*

I read Psalm 91 in the Bible Celia has lent me, then in the version that Juliet has given me, and then in my own Bible, and I'm struck by the variations in the text. They all hold to the same core but they are different versions.

As a publisher and editor, I'm aware of how powerful even minor changes in text can be, how nuances of words and rhythms can change the impact of what is written. I look at the different versions of this Psalm and others, and I think that no text is absolute. The sacred word has been adapted for thousands of years, in different translations, revisions, new

245

editions, highlighting or emphasising certain aspects according to the theology and needs of those doing the revision.

A line from Psalm 46 hits me: '*God is in that city; she will not be overthrown*', and although it becomes clear that the 'she' refers to the city, I'm struck by the power of the feminine pronoun.

I've read that in the ancient Hebrew of the Psalms there are no gender-specific pronouns and that God is above the concept of gender in the Judaic tradition, and I start to adapt some of the psalms myself, particularly the pronouns, looking for more inclusive terminology, looking for the 'She'. I arrive at my version of that part of Psalm 46:

God is in the world
She will not be overthrown
And She will help us at the break of day.

Sitting upstairs in my study, reading, I hear Peter's car return from the embassy. I hear him enter the house, look at my watch and see it's lunchtime already. I close my book and go downstairs to greet him.

'Hi, sweetheart,' I say and give him a kiss. 'How was your morning?'

'OK,' he says. He puts his briefcase down in his study, leads me into the sitting room, and sits down on the sofa. I sit beside him.

'I got a call from the President today,' he tells me.

I look more closely at him.

'Is he telling us we're on the move again?' I ask, jokingly.

'How did you know?' asks Peter, looking surprised.

'No! I didn't know. I'm playing. You're not serious, are you?' I splutter.

'I am,' he says. 'The President is reassigning me.'

'Oh, my God!' I say. 'Where?'

'Berlin,' says Peter.

I don't know what to say. This is completely unexpected. Peter was appointed for four years to his post in Brussels and we thought we had two more years to go, and that we would return to a quiet life in Namibia after that.

'How long have we got?' I ask Peter.

'The President has submitted my name to the Germans and we have to wait for them to accept,' he says, 'but we'll have to start packing soon.'

'And who will come here?'

'The current Ambassador in Berlin.'

'So you're just swapping over?'

'Yes.'

The thought of all this move will entail makes me decide not to proceed with the operation to put in a new pacemaker; I can't cope with that as well.

'Oh, no!' Isabel says, when we tell her. 'I can't believe it! Not a second time!'

Once again, our move will pull Isabel out of her school and the circle of friends she's now found. She has one more year of school left, to finish her A-levels; it's not a good time to change schools.

We search through the websites of international schools in Berlin looking for a school for her to transfer to, but find none that offer the same A-level courses Isabel is studying.

'I think she'll have to stay in Brussels to finish her A-levels,' I say to Peter, 'and I'll have to find a way to stay with her while you go to Berlin. Or we could try to find a host family for her.'

This time, however, Isabel takes charge. She has already started to look at different universities and courses, encouraged by the school to start to think about these things, in anticipation of applying next year. She looks at American universities in Europe, some of which come to the school to address the pupils, and she finds a course at one that interests her – International Relations – at a satellite campus of an American university in the ancient university city of Leiden, in The Netherlands. Since it is in the American education system, Isabel is eligible to start after the AS-level exams that she has just completed. She applies and is accepted, and she gets a small scholarship based on her application essay. She prepares to start in August and is allocated a room in a flat, which she will share with other students.

Then follows the farewell process: weeks of packing and partying and (in my case) praying. I face each day as it comes, unsure of what the future holds, sad to be leaving Brussels at the point when Peter and I really feel we know what we are doing, sad that we will not see the places we had intended to visit, nor complete some of the projects with which we were involved and sad to leave the women I've come to know. I'm also nervous about what Berlin will be like. Lingering prejudices against Germany come to the surface from deep in my English upbringing, plus anxiety about Isabel leaving school and home a year earlier than we anticipated, and the knowledge that I will have to look for a new cardiologist in Berlin and face the question of getting a new pacemaker there.

There is a particular ring of Brigitte's that I like, with a dark blue stone, which Tobi gave me after she died. I name it Brigitte's 'ring of courage' and I put it on each day to give me courage too.

This time, the move happens all too fast. We load up the removal truck in Brussels and race to Berlin to join it there, then must immediately unpack and start sorting our belongings and getting them into some semblance of order in our new house.

I begin to understand Peter's non-attachment to houses – he has moved so many times in his life, especially during the years of the liberation struggle. Each time, he unpacks his clothes and his papers and gets on with his work. The arranging of furniture, artwork, ornaments, books, etc. are my domain, as I try to make the place a home.

The house in Berlin is squarer than the one in Brussels and close to the road, although it's a small, tree-lined, cobbled side-street. We have neighbours nearby on each side, and after the huge surrounding garden we had in Brussels, it's strange to hear the occasional noises of people next door. There are three floors and a basement, with a flat in which the cook/housekeeper, Lambert, his wife Janet, and young daughter Jesse, live. On the ground floor is a huge open-plan reception room with a long, highly polished, wooden table in the dining area, and nine sofas arranged in two sitting areas. There's pale yellow material on the walls; we're told not to knock in any nails to hang our artwork there, because it is French silk.

Our bedroom is on the first floor, as well as a guest bedroom and large family room, which is a cold, impersonal place with grey walls, plain white net curtains, a dark green marble fireplace and shelf and dark brown leather chairs. It's a challenge to think of ways of making it look warmer and feel more comfortable without a budget for paint or furnishings.

There are two bedrooms at the top, under the eaves, for Perivi and Isabel, when they are with us, and a large room that Peter and I decide to share as a study, all with white walls, wooden beams and windows angled into the roof. It's the only floor that feels like private, as opposed to public, space.

The small front garden is filled with low green bushes and a large magnolia tree. The main garden, at the back, is a quarter the size of the one in Brussels but more user-friendly. It has large trees around one side, including two of the plane trees that are common in Berlin, a swimming pool, summer house, and a wooden bench in a corner under silver birch trees, with bamboo growing round it.

The day after we finish unpacking, dull chest pains wake me in the middle of the night. I tell myself it's just tiredness after the move but the pain comes and goes and I drift in and out of sleep. In the morning, I tell Peter.

'Just rest today,' he says. 'You've been doing a lot. Get Lambert to help you.'

I spend the day reading and hope that will help. That night, I sleep through with no problems, but the next day I have repeated runs of rapid heartbeats in the afternoon. I try to breathe deeply to calm my heart but the speed of the heartbeats takes my breath away and makes me feel dizzy. Each run passes after a few seconds but they keep coming. After about 15 minutes, when the rapid heartbeats stop, I phone Peter. He asks the embassy for advice about doctors and they recommend a cardiologist who's looked after many Namibians in the past. They phone and make an appointment for me for the next day.

In the morning, Edward, the driver, comes to collect us. He's tall and thin, from Benin, and is also a pastor of a Pentecostal church. He drives Peter and me east across this formerly divided city to find the surgery. We travel for nearly an hour, through the shopping streets of the old centre of West Berlin, the building sites in East Berlin, down Karl-Marx-Allee, a long, wide, boulevard built in the 1950s. It's lined on both sides with heavy eight-storey buildings and was the site of the annual May Day parade in the days of the GDR.

'I didn't know it was so far,' I say. 'It feels as if we're going to Poland.' The border is only an hour's drive from Berlin.

We find the door to the surgery, at the side of a pharmacy, and go up to the second floor in the lift. The waiting room is light and has modern abstract paintings on the wall. About ten people are waiting but we're seen almost straight away. The cardiologist comes down the corridor personally to greet us.

'Ambassador, come in please.'

He tells us of his past involvement with solidarity work in support of Namibia and some of the Namibians he has seen, including both President Nujoma and his wife, on past visits of theirs to Berlin. Then he asks me about my problems.

I have a medical report from the cardiologist in Brussels, which I give him, and I explain the symptoms of the previous few days. He listens to my heart and does a sonar and an ECG.

'I want to find out more about what's happening with your heart,' he tells me. 'Can you come back on Friday and we can arrange a portable monitor for you?'

We go back to the residence and I spend the next day listlessly, wondering what the monitor will show this time, but glad it's something I can wear at home, so I don't have to go into hospital. When I return to the surgery on Friday morning, the cardiologist attaches electrodes to my chest that connect to a monitor the size of a cassette recorder, which is then tucked into a little bag with a string to hold it round my neck. He advises me to wear a vest that will hold the wires close to my body so the electrodes don't come off.

I'm anxious that I won't be able to sleep that night with the monitor on, but I find that I can lie partly on one side, with a pillow propped behind my back. It's fine until I try to turn over, then I become aware of the monitor, wake up and have to rearrange myself. In the morning, I run a very shallow bath, climb in, and wash myself carefully with a flannel, avoiding the wires and electrodes. I potter round the house during the next two days, wondering where to hang our artwork and put our ornaments. I try out the different sofas downstairs, with their views of the back or front garden, put my feet up, and read. I go up to the family room and turn on the TV to see if there's anything to watch, but discover that all the channels are in German. After three days, I unplug the electrodes myself and give the monitor to Edward to take back.

'I've looked at the results, Mrs Katjavivi,' the cardiologist tells me when Peter and I go for my follow-up appointment. 'I don't think there's enough evidence of tachycardia to need a new pacemaker.'

'Really?' I ask, surprised.

'Yes,' he says. 'I was at a conference recently that looked at treatment for your condition, and I've discussed your case with a colleague as well. The latest thinking in Germany is to treat your condition with medication unless it gets much worse. Only then might you need a different type of pacemaker.'

'I'm so relieved,' I tell him. 'Thank you.'

He changes some of the medication I take and adjusts the doses.

'Imagine if we hadn't come to Berlin,' I say to Peter on the way back in the car. 'I'd have probably had that operation.'

'I'm so glad you don't need to.'

Freed from the anxiety about having a radically different pacemaker, and with the intensity of the move behind me, I start to unwind. It's late summer, and the diplomatic season has not yet started, so there are no lunches or dinners to go to; nothing is expected of me.

I take the time to rest at home. The corner of the garden under the silver birch trees becomes my sacred place. I sit there quietly, the breeze blowing the leaves on the trees, and calm descends. I read or pray or write and I explore what I believe. As autumn advances and the leaves fall, I read about Christianity, Buddhism and Islam. I look at a collection of wise thoughts from African prophets that we bought in Brussels and am particularly fond of one from Birago Diop:

> Listen more often
> To things than to people.
> The voice of the fire can be heard
> Hear the voice of the water
> Listen to the wind
> The sobbing bush:
> It is the sigh of the ancestors...

As the weather gets colder, I move inside and read about the origin of the pyramids and ancient belief systems from different cultures across the world. I take comfort in devotional words and religious revelation from different faiths.

From Judaism, the Psalms and the ancient tradition of the prophets. From Islam, the simple statement of faith: there is one God. From Christianity, the message of love, redemption and healing. From African tradition, the recognition that the spirit is the force, the life that is found in everything. From Buddhism the elemental connection between all living things: the 'I' that is 'We'. From Hinduism, the wondrous revelation that 'God is one and has a million faces,' and recognition of duality in the goddess Kali – god of creation and destruction.

I mark the writings that speak to me and collect a pile of books on my bedside table, waiting for me to copy out the parts I like. I start a notebook with my own thoughts, and prayers and lines from my favourite Psalms. I start my own statement of faith:

I believe in God, Father and Mother of the universe,
Maker of all things, visible and invisible,
The source of love,
On whom we can call for protection
To strengthen ourselves
And find our way in the world.

I believe in the Absolute, the Creator,
The source of energy and light and life,
The spirit that is within all living things,
In which we are One,
Who has many faces and many names.

I believe that I am part of something bigger than myself,
A part of Life, a part of creation.
I believe that we are Fire and Water,
Yin and Yan,
Creator and Destroyer,
And that the life force of which we are part
Has those same characteristics of opposites,
Like lightning, like electricity,
Cracking across the universe,
Creating/giving life,
Destroying/burning,
Burning/healing.

I believe
That we acknowledge and recognise the life force
And give it different names
At different historical ages,
In different times.
Across time and culture,
We make the connection,
We search for the pattern and the meaning,
And we call this God.

This is my time of reflection and revelation. In the still spaces of the night and in early waking moments, comes knowledge beyond the everyday consciousness. I come to know that I am part of the collective heartbeat. I come to terms with my beginning and my end. I come to terms with the death of the body. I stop being afraid.

Isabel settles well into student life in Leiden. She loves the canals and the small cobbled streets down which she cycles to class. She enjoys the courses she's taking and her new independent existence, sharing a flat with two visiting American students and cooking for herself. Perivi is much happier at the film school in Los Angeles, and is busy getting into the practicalities of film production, and writing scripts – Namibian stories – for future films.

Our lives take on a different rhythm, particularly mine, because both children have now flown. Peter rarely comes back for lunch as the residence is further from the embassy than it was in Brussels, so I'm on my own much of the day. Time has a different quality. I am largely left to my own devices. I sort through my papers, finding notes I've made, and I start to write. I write about my friends in Namibia and our health crises, trying to understand what happened to us. I write about the upheaval of going to Brussels and learning how to cope with diplomatic life.

Our residence is in Dahlem, a middle-class area with many university people and students, as the Free University of Berlin is nearby. There are large detached houses and tree-lined streets, and the Botanical Gardens are five minutes from the house. In the evenings, Peter and I go for walks round the area. At weekends, we walk through the Botanical Gardens. Sometimes we end up at a small Italian restaurant or a beer garden nearby. We have more time together. We're free to go by the underground U-Bahn to a film on the spur of the moment, or by car or bus to the shopping area of Steglitz, which is not far away, and spend the afternoon in the bookshop, browsing without any obligation to buy. To put classical music on loud so that it reverberates through the house, or watch football on TV. To spread the Sunday newspapers across the coffee table and read them all afternoon, until Peter puts his head on my knee when he gets sleepy and I give him a head massage.

Peter does the rounds of embassies to introduce himself to other ambassadors. He is immediately taken up with work at the embassy and meetings with German politicians and businessmen. I gradually join the women's networks, as I did in Brussels.

There's an Association of Spouses of African Ambassadors – smaller than the ACP spouses group, and not including all the African embassies as some have not yet moved from the old German capital, Bonn. The first of their monthly lunches I attend is at the Egyptian residence. Only nine women are there, and half of us are new. We introduce ourselves: name, profession, diplomatic postings, number of children, interests.

'I was in the ACP Spouses group in Brussels,' I tell them, 'and we did a lot of fund-raising work,' but I downplay my role. They are looking for new committee members and I don't want to take on any new responsibilities.

We move into the dining room for a light buffet lunch. The conversation is dominated by two very talkative women who've been in Berlin for some years and who tell the rest of us about the diplomatic community there and who is who.

'You must get involved,' the new arrivals are told. 'We need to build up the group and make it stronger.'

I miss the Caribbean and Pacific members who were also part of our association in Brussels and when I get home, I send a joint email to the members of the gala committee, to tell them about the lunch and bring them up to date about how we are doing and how my health is.

'I've found a really nice cardiologist who's keeping an eye on me and has changed my medication to try to calm down my dancing heart,' I write. 'I'm trying to stay calm and be positive and connect with God and the universe and encourage my heart to sing rather than to dance.'

I also join Wilkommen in Berlin, which is open to spouses of all diplomats, not just ambassadors. It's a large group with a wide range of activities, started by wives of German diplomats when the Government and Foreign Ministry moved to Berlin, to help diplomatic spouses from other countries, and to help themselves since they were also new to the city. Through this group, I meet German women; they are less formal than the Belgian women I met, and more direct, which I enjoy.

Peter and I start German classes at the Goethe Institut in the eastern part of Berlin. Different teachers teach us individually but our classes are at the same time. Peter has picked up some German from his childhood in Namibia and through contacts with German friends and acquaintances over the years. I discover there's a door in my memory to the German I learnt at school but never used.

We leave straight after breakfast, and practice our German on each other.

'*Mein liebling, bist du vertig?* – Are you ready, darling?' I ask Peter as we leave the breakfast table and pick up our bags.

'*Naturlich,*' he replies.

'*Um wieviel Uhr kommst du nach Hause heute?* – What time are you coming home today?' I ask.

'*Nicht zu spat* – Not too late.'

Because of the different way we've learnt the language, I know the structure quite well, but Peter's understanding is better than mine.

The trip to and from the Goethe Institut, and the class itself, take up most of the morning, and after a few months, Peter has to stop his classes because of his work commitments. I find the morning journey difficult because my blood pressure goes down after I take my medication, and I'm tired for a couple of hours before my body absorbs it. I arrange, therefore, for my German teacher, Elisabeth, to come to the residence twice a week to continue my lessons. We go upstairs to the family room, sit at a small table there, and talk about a range of topics, from hairdressers to newspaper reports she finds for me to read, or issues I want to discuss. She's younger than me, in her late thirties or early forties, I estimate, with a young son. I get on with very well with her and think she may become a friend, until her husband is appointed as the German Ambassador to Yemen and they leave Berlin.

There are old friends and connections here, who supported Namibia's liberation struggle: people from the former East Germany and the former West – trade unionists, politicians, churchmen and women, and NGO activists. The second in command at the South African embassy is an old friend from our London days, who worked with the ANC Youth League and with SWAPO there. He takes us out to dinner soon after we arrive, to Gendarmenmarkt, Berlin's most beautiful square. It has a concert hall and two domed cathedrals – the 'French' one built by Huguenot refugees in the early eighteenth century and a 'German' one built later in similar style. We talk about the past of the liberation movement and the present diplomatic world that he and Peter both inhabit. I raise my glass to them:

'I want to toast the two of you and your achievements, both personal and political,' I say. 'Who would have thought when we were working together in London that we would be here one day?'

There are more Namibians in Germany than in most other European countries, and quite a few in Berlin, who provide us with an immediate community: people who came to study before Independence and stayed on, those who have come to work here for a while, and those who have married and settled in Germany, as did Luther.

There's also direct family: Uazuvara's daughter Aicha, born while Uazuvara was living here in the 1970s with his Zimbabwean wife, and her 12-year-old son Kara; Luther's daughter, Miriam, who used to come and stay with us in Windhoek, her husband Matthias and their two little girls.

Miriam and Matthias take us on a tour of the city in an open-topped bus. They both grew up in East Germany and don't know the former West Berlin very well, so they are discovering the city as are we. They have two girls, named after Sandra and Mosé's daughters. The older, Paulina Tjireya, is a bright, lively, two-year-old who already talks in complete sentences, describing her emotions and telling her parents what she needs. The younger, Carlotta Ripuree, is born a few months after we arrive in Berlin. She has a difficult start to life with some medical complications. Happily, these are resolved and I have the joy of becoming her godmother at a ceremony in the church where her parents were married, in Ludwigslust in north-eastern Germany.

Edward drives us to Ludwigslust, through the flat lands and past the lakes of Mecklenburg-Vorpommern, Germany's least-populated state. Its northern Baltic coast is popular with tourists. Its capital, Schwerin, is where some 400 Namibian children were looked after and educated in the 1980s.

The Lutheran church in Ludwigslust is square, with dusky pink walls and columns. Inside, the walls are white-washed and devoid of decoration except for a huge mural in the circular enclave behind the altar. I join Miriam and Matthias, the girls and the other godparents in front of the altar for the baptismal vows. Miriam and Matthias have chosen a Bible text for each of their daughters, to guide them in life. Carlotta's is 1 Corinthians 13, verse 7:

'There is nothing love cannot face; there is no limit to its faith, its hope, and its endurance.'

Uazuvara's daughter, Aicha, is tall, with a broad chest and shoulders, just like her father. She's full of energy, talkative, understanding, immediately sensing what is going on with people and situations, which is also like her father. To my surprise, she remembers me from the time I first visited Berlin 30 years ago, when she was just a child, and she tells me that I haven't changed. We connect immediately and arrange to meet for coffee at the Literary Society café just off Kurfurstendamm. It's near Aicha's flat, in the very centre of the former West Berlin. The café is on the first floor of a large semi-detached stone house with a garden. There's a small bookshop on the garden level, and a programme of talks and poetry readings. We sit in the glass-covered terrace at the top of the steps leading up to the café, and I order Earl Grey tea. Aicha has black coffee.

'So Aicha,' I say, 'your father tells me you are Super Mama.' She has worked with children for many years and recently starred in a television reality show of that name, in which she advised families on how to look after difficult or misbehaving children.

Aicha laughs. 'It was hard work,' she says, 'looking after the children and the parents, and all the time with the television filming. But the series has ended.'

'What are you doing now?' I ask her and she tells me about her work with children taken from situations of danger, who need urgent care.

'They come into the home I'm working in,' she says, 'and then later they will go on to foster families.'

'It must be draining emotionally,' I say.

'Yes. There are some children in terrible situations. You can't believe what some people do to their children.'

The waitress comes and asks us if we want anything else, but we decline. After she's gone, Aicha turns the conversation to our family:

'Tell me more about Isabel and Perivi,' she says and I explain what they are doing.

'Tell me more about Jane,' she says, and I pour my heart out to her.

'Talking to Aicha is like taking a truth serum,' I tell Peter when he gets home that evening. 'I thought we were just going to have coffee, but I ended up telling her all about myself.'

I ask Aicha if she can recommend a hairdresser for Isabel when she visits. In Brussels, she went to the African area of Matonge to get her hair done but we have searched unsuccessfully for an African hairdresser in Berlin. The one Aicha recommends is called 'Ebony and Ivory' and advertises that it does African and European hair. When I take Isabel there during one of her visits, there are a number of stylists at work. On one side of the salon are a couple of young black men doing sharp razor cuts for black and white male customers. On the other side are the women — one white and three black stylists, and six young brown women who are having their hair done. It makes me feel at home.

With members of the family in Berlin, I don't feel an urgent need to find new friends. I also keep the rest of the extended family close, through photos that I place along the heavy marble shelf of the family room in the residence. They greet us each day as we walk in. My parents, my sisters, Peter as a young man, his mother and his Aunt Maria, my grandfather, our children and grandchildren. My favourite photo is one I took at Miriam and Matthias's wedding. It is of Miriam's side of the family and includes her mother Gisela, her two fathers (Luther and Erich, who brought her up), her sisters and their boyfriends, her brother (Luther's son but not Gisela's) with his partner and their baby son. Luther's new partner Evelin, Brigitte's son Tobi and his partner, Patji, Egil and Isabel are also there. All in one glorious mosaic.

I no longer look at relatives the English way. Cousins are brothers and sisters; aunts are mothers and uncles are fathers, as in Namibia. I don't count the stages of removal that are so clearly defined in England. For me there are no steps or halves: all our children are whole.

When I came to Berlin 30 years ago, I visited Uazuvara and he took me to see the ruined Gedächtniskirche at the end of Kurfurstendamm, with bullet holes in the walls. It was a shock to me, coming from England. I had grown up with stories of British cities bombed by the Germans but the damage was not as extensive as the British and American bombing of German cities in the late stages of the war. The damage to British cities, moreover, did not include bullet holes – the legacy of soldiers fighting it out in the streets.

I remember thinking, back then, that Berlin was a city of ghosts, that nothing was named. Now, we find that there are names and memorials everywhere. Outside the Reichstag is a memorial to the Members of Parliament executed by the Nazis. Round the corner, towards the Brandenburg Gate, and on bridges over the river, are photographs and/ or crosses commemorating people shot while trying to cross the Wall from East to West Berlin. Small segments of the Wall remain in places, and a cobbled marker on the ground traces the path it took.

Beyond the Brandenburg Gate is the new Memorial for the Murdered Jews of Europe, an impressive commemoration of the darkest days of Germany's history, with an underground information centre giving the names of all known Holocaust victims. Round the corner again, in the Tiergarten Park, is a memorial to the Soviet soldiers killed liberating Berlin. Around the city, individual brass cobbles appear at our feet outside restaurants and shops, with names on them of people who were dragged from their homes there and sent to the concentration camps in the Nazi period.

The Memorial for the Murdered Jews of Europe is composed of sculpted concrete blocks of different heights that form alleyways criss-crossing each other in rigid lines. I go there with an old friend, Jo, who worked with the Namibia Support Committee in London in the 1970s, and knew Peter before I did. I remember being very impressed when I first knew her because she pushed her young son Daniel in a stroller on anti-apartheid demonstrations. She works now for the Trade Union Congress in London on equality and women's employment rights and comes to Berlin for a meeting with the German Confederation of Trade Unions. She stays on for a couple of days to see us.

Jo and I walk through the pathways between the concrete blocks on the sloping Memorial site. Where the land dips, the blocks rise high above us, cold to the touch, and forbidding. They shut out the sounds of the city beyond. I turn one way and then another and Jo goes a different way. We quickly get lost. It feels as if there is no escape.

A few discreetly placed security guards make sure that people respect the site and don't throw litter or play games there. There's no graffiti, and we read from the information provided that the stones of the blocks are coated with special chemicals to resist the paint of graffiti. The chemicals are appropriately made by the very company that produced the gas for the gas chambers in the 1940s.

After visiting the Memorial, we walk across to Potsdamer Platz, a newly developed complex with restaurants and cinemas. We sit at an outside table of one of its many cafés, and have a coffee. Jo looks up at the conical glass roof and the dramatic modern buildings around Potsdamer Platz. She's an enthusiastic person who engages with everything around her.

'I really like Berlin,' she says. 'There's a lot going on.'

'Yes, there's a lot of energy here.' I reply. 'And we keep bumping into political history. It keeps me aware of the important issues, rather like being in Southern Africa,' I add.

We move on again to Museum Island, literally an island in the River Spree in the old historical centre of Berlin; it's a UNESCO World Heritage Site. We go into the Pergamon Museum, named after the enormous altar from the ancient Greek temple at Pergamon, which it houses. We walk round the carved frieze of life-size human and mythical figures, and up the steps to the columns of the altar. We descend again and pass into another room and then through an arched gateway. A large sign instructs us to turn round and we do so. We see that we've just walked through the reconstructed gate of the ancient city of Babylon, covered with blue and amber tiles, many of them originals, and with large golden lions prancing across it. The lions continue along a blue-tiled causeway that leads up to the gate.

'I'm amazed,' I say to Jo, and then confess, 'I realise that I've always regarded Babylon as a mythical, not a real city.'

We go into the other rooms of the museum and discover other artefacts from Babylon, plus Syrian and Mesopotamian statues, wall friezes and a model of the Tower of Babel based on measurements taken during an archaeological dig at the site of Babylon.

'You know, in principle I don't approve of the expropriation of national cultural treasures such as these.' I say. 'But I delight in this opportunity to see them.'

A persistent question Peter and I and other newcomers have is whether something is in the former East or former West of the city. Sometimes we can recognise that we've crossed the old line of the Wall by the state of the buildings. Parts of the former East have been renovated and rebuilt but other areas still look poor in comparison with those in the former West, and the buildings are often covered with graffiti.

'The West spent their money on buildings,' said Matthias when we went on the bus tour together and could see these differences. 'The GDR spent its money on people.'

Now, Berlin is spending money on renovating the former East and there are too many demands on the city's budget.

'I get confused about directions here,' Jo told me when she was visiting. 'And I didn't expect the Wall to meander through the city the way it did.'

'I know,' I replied. 'I thought that East Germany was simply east of the Wall, but now I realise that the East was also north and south and west of West Berlin. I didn't really appreciate until now that West Berlin was the oddity, the island surrounded by "East" Germany.'

When two other old friends from England, Judith and Terry, come to visit, I take them on a circular tour to try to show this to them. We start at the residence and go west at first, through the nearby Grunewald Forest and round its lake, where people walk and picnic on the small beaches. Some of the spots are reserved for nudists, as Peter and I discovered when we walked there one weekend.

We drive round the north side of the lake to the Luftwaffe Museum, which Terry wants to visit because he's interested in old aeroplanes, and we drop him there. Judith and I then head south into what used to be East Germany. We pass through villages that look as if they haven't changed for decades and stop at Potsdam, where the conference at the end of the Second World War was held.

'We could visit the Palace of Sans Souci,' I suggest to Judith. It's a seat of the Prussian kings and has been expensively redone, attracting large numbers of tourists.

I haven't seen Judith and Terry for over ten years and wasn't sure what they would like to do. But Judith has been involved in community development, housing and health provision for most of her professional life.

'I'm more interested in seeing Potsdam itself,' she tells me and we drive into the town and find somewhere to park. We walk round the old seventeenth century centre that is slowly being renovated, find a café and sit down for a cup of coffee.

'It's so nice, just being with you like this and picking up as if we'd seen you regularly,' Judith says, smiling. She has thick brown hair, rosy cheeks and a warm manner.

'I know,' I reply. She is a friend from my early days in London, before I met Peter, but I saw her only rarely after I became involved in work on Southern Africa.

'Do you remember our holiday in Greece?' I ask her. A group of us had rented a villa on Kos in the late 1970s, and travelled round the island on rented motorbikes.

'Yes, I still remember it,' Judith says.

'It was when we were on Kos that I realised I was in love with Peter,' I tell her. She is intrigued.

'Tell me more,' she says.

'Peter was in Angola at the time for a SWAPO Central Committee meeting, and I was always worried about him when he was in Angola,' I explain. 'I remember that every day we were in Greece, when we came back to the villa from the beach or from a trip, I would see something white under the vase of flowers on the table as I walked up to the house. I always thought it was a telegram telling me that something terrible had happened to Peter, but it was only a paper napkin placed under the vase.' I pause. 'I realised then that if I thought about him that much all the time, even when I was on holiday, it was a sign of how much I loved him. It sort of crept up on me.'

Judith takes a drink of her coffee. 'Terry and I weren't surprised when you told me you and Peter were together,' she says. 'You talked about him all the time.'

We finish our coffee, return to the car, and go to pick up Terry. Then we head east again into what was West Berlin, coming round the southern tip of the Wahnsee Lake, to the bridge where prisoners were exchanged during the Cold War. We pass expensive yachts in beautiful

264

marinas and the most expensive houses in the city. We come to the lakeside villa where the Wahnsee conference took place in 1942. This was the place where the plans for the systematic extermination of the Jews were drawn up.

'I think we have to stop here,' says Terry and we go inside.

A written record of the conference proceedings has been found that shows how the heads of different government and military departments competed to offer a final solution. A young guide takes us through the detail of who said what. Chilled after hearing all of this, and in the growing darkness, we drive back through forest towards our home. Wild boars run out of the trees ahead of us and we have to brake to avoid them. They are like the warthogs in Namibia, only thicker set at the shoulder and with shorter tusks.

We were blessed in Brussels by visits from family and friends and so we are in Berlin too. My parents come to visit us, despite their misgivings about Germany, having had their adult lives shaped by the fight against fascism in the Second World War. I decide to go to England to see them first, and bring them back with me to Berlin.

'I want to take my parents on a tour of the city,' I tell Edward once we have returned. 'But I don't want them to see the Reichstag.'

'Why, Madame?' he asks, looking curious.

'I don't want to remind them of the Nazi past,' I say. 'Can we take them round the back somehow?'

'Yes, Madame,' he says and he drives us round Potsdamer Platz and cuts across to Unten den Linden, one of the famous avenues of Berlin before the war that was cut in half by the Wall.

We have tea in the luxurious lounge of the Adlon Hotel, and sit in large comfortable armchairs while a pianist plays gentle music in one corner. When we've finished our tea, we walk out of the hotel and turn to our left. The Brandenburg Gate is 100 metres in front of us, standing astride the street, its pale sandstone structure cleaned and a bronze statue of the goddess of victory on the top.

'Let's just go up to the Gate itself,' I say to my parents. But I've forgotten that the Reichstag is so near the Gate and the moment we get there, we can see it. Contrary to my expectations, my parents are interested.

I have memories of black and white Nazi propaganda films showing Hitler standing in front of the Reichstag with thousands of supporters spread out across the square in front, swastika flags flying, arms raised in the Nazi salute, and I've always associated the building with Hitler. It is not until coming to Berlin that I realise that the Reichstag was not Hitler's seat of government. A fire started there in February 1933 and rendered the building unusable. It provided an excuse for the government to declare a state of emergency and round up those opposed to the regime, and led to the installation of the National Socialist dictatorship. It's generally accepted that the fire was set by the Nazis themselves. The burning of the Reichstag in 1933 was therefore seen as a violent act against democracy. The renovation and reopening of it in 1999 to house the current Parliament of a unified Germany has been a reassertion of democracy.

More usually, our tour for visitors starts with a boat trip that goes through the different parts of the city – east and west, historical and modern, residential and industrial. We take my parents on a boat tour, my sister Sarah and her husband Dennis, and Uanaingi, when she comes to visit with her nine-year-old daughter Utaa, while Isabel is at home on vacation. We think of things Utaa might like to do and Isabel encourages us to take them to the zoo. She wants to come as well, even though as a child she was able to visit Etosha and other Namibian national parks and see animals in the wild. I'm not keen on the idea of visiting caged animals but the zoo is a large, open, green space in the centre of Berlin, and it's wonderful for children.

'I love seeing the gorillas and tigers – animals I haven't seen before,' I confess to Isabel as we go round the zoo. 'But it's distressing to see large animals – buffalo, elephant, giraffe, rhino and lions – in small enclosures.'

'They look so sad,' she agrees.

The delight for Utaa is seeing Knut, a polar bear cub born at the zoo and raised by zookeepers after he was rejected by his mother. He's the first polar bear cub to survive past infancy at the Berlin Zoo in more than 30 years. We queue for an hour to see Knut, playing games with Utaa to keep her from getting bored. Peter carries her on his shoulders and tells her stories about jackals that he was told as a child. Isabel takes her to one of the playgrounds while we keep our place in the queue. We get ice-creams and drinks to keep us going.

When we reach the polar bear enclosure, we have to keep to a path and are told by zoo staff to keep moving because there are so many people wanting to see Knut. We look across an area of water to a rocky island behind, and Knut walks out of a small cave mouth, as if on cue, and looks across at us. He's about the height of a German Shepherd dog, but fluffy and white and very cute. The keeper comes in and waves a blanket at Knut, to attract his attention. He plays with him for a while, and we move on out of the enclosure.

The zoo is also a favourite place for Patji's children, Egil and Meri, when they come. During one of their visits, we have a delightful coming together of family and friends. My parents are with us, Patji and the children (Heidi is in Finland with her parents), a nephew from Namibia, and Nita and her husband Aachim, who are in Berlin for business.

Egil and Meri eat in the kitchen and go downstairs afterwards to watch television with Lambert's daughter Jesse. The adults sit around our long dining room table and enjoy a dinner Lambert has prepared for us. We talk about international politics, and our nephew makes a negative comment about 'mad Muslims'.

'You can't talk like that about people,' I tell him from across the table.

'But they're the ones causing all the trouble in the world.'

'Please,' I say, 'don't make those generalisations. We have someone who's a Muslim with us at the table tonight,' thinking of Nita but not wanting to draw direct attention to her.

'I don't like Muslims,' he says, 'or Catholics.'

'Stop it, please!' I say. I pick up my table napkin and throw it across the table at him. It doesn't quite reach him but lands on a plate nearby. The others have gone silent and we continue eating.

'I found out something very interesting about my family background not so long ago,' says Aachim after a while. 'I discovered that my grandmother spent some time in Russia, and had a relationship with a Russian Jew while she was there. She fell pregnant and was hastily brought home by her parents, and married to a German. The child and subsequent grandchildren, including me, were brought up as Christians.'

He has caught our attention and we all listen to his story. 'Nita is Muslim,' he affirms, 'and I'm very proud to have these three great religions – Judaism, Christianity and Islam – in the family.'

Soon afterwards, Deedee and Michael also visit us, with Deedee's parents. They arrive by boat, coming from the Czech Republic, at the end of a cruise down the River Elbe; it's an 80th birthday celebration for Deedee's mother. They stay with us for a couple of days after their tour is over. Deedee's mother is an energetic and gracious woman with the soft accent of the American South. Her grey hair is slightly wavy. Her smile is generous and her mind is quick, like Deedee's. They go together to all the museums on Museum Island, as does Michael. Deedee's father and I take things at a slower pace.

Deedee's father is a retired university professor, her mother a former history teacher, and they travel widely. They visit countries outside the normal tourist routes, including Iran in the early 1990s; and they recently went on a skiing holiday even though they're in their eighties

My parents are also in their eighties, and Jane's father is 99. He last visited her in Namibia when he was 96, staying for three months or so through the hottest months of the year, spending a lot of time with her son Freddie, then a young teenager.

'He's frail but very charming, elegant and easy,' Deedee tells me. Sadly, I've never met him.

'You know, I have to tell you about Helao,' Deedee says. 'He's been made a colonel, honoured by President Pohamba, and given a medal at last year's commemoration of the launching of the armed struggle.'

'Really?' I ask. 'I missed that completely.'

'No, it's wonderful,' Deedee says. 'And Jane was so delighted. We're all delighted that his contribution to the struggle has finally been publicly acknowledged in this way. And it was a very special commemoration because it was the 40th anniversary of the launching of the armed struggle.'

'What was the ceremony like?' I ask.

'Well, Jane told us about it at Friday breakfast. It was one of the best moments of Friday breakfast, I tell you. But Jane herself missed the ceremony because Freddie was suddenly taken ill and she had to take him to the doctor!'

Representing Namibia in Germany is very different from doing so in Belgium. Here people know about and are interested in the country. Some have old family connections; others love to visit Namibia, where they can speak German much of the time in hotels, restaurants and shops.

The challenge for the embassy is to respond to the interest and try to channel it into tourism, investment or development support. It means that Peter is very busy once again, and he travels off to meetings four hours away by road rather than the shorter distances we got used to in Belgium.

Peter embarks on a series of visits to towns in different German states, and I go with him, able to do so more easily now that I don't need to worry about leaving Isabel. We get to know more about the country and the people, build connections, and try to encourage investment and cultural exchange. We discover people here who spend more time in Namibia than we do; going there three or four times a year, and keen to talk about their visits.

Berlin is partnered with Windhoek, despite the difference in the sizes of the cities. The mayors of the two towns have visited each other's cities. There have been cultural visits and exchanges, and one of the Members of the Berlin State Parliament teams up with a visiting Namibian artist to develop a programme to support cultural exchange between the two cities.

There is a German Namibia Society with members from all over Germany, who hold meetings on Namibia and raise funds for specific projects, including another cultural exchange programme. The Chairperson, Klaus, is a publisher I've known for many years. He published a German edition of a book about the Namibian children schooled in the GDR, when I published the English version. Rudiger and Frauke, both doctors, and members of the Society, come to the residence one weekend to discuss a fund-raising event for the Ombili Foundation, that supports a San community in north-central Namibia. I make a cup of tea for us all and we sit around one of the coffee tables in our large reception room.

'We have two big functions every year,' Rudi tells us. 'One is a festival in the park. We sell the tickets and we cook a big meal.'

'Who does the cooking?' I ask.

'Everyone on the committee joins in,' he says. 'But Frauke and I, we love to cook.' Rudi is quite round. His wife Frauke is petite and slim, with very short, wavy grey hair. Both are full of enthusiasm for the project.

'What we want to know,' Frauke says, 'is whether your cook could give us advice about cooking African food for our festival this year.'

'I'm sure he'd love to,' I reply. I talk to Lambert about it later and Rudi and Frauke come to meet him and plan the meal directly. When the time for the festival arrives, they come to the residence very early in the morning and work with Lambert to prepare the food for their event.

Food preparation plays a large part in my life, although it's Lambert who does most of the actual work.

We host a Namibian Sunday brunch in Berlin at a restaurant in a converted light-bulb factory. It's part of a series of monthly networking brunches with different country themes organised by Michael, a journalist we get to know. He puts our lunch down on the list at short notice and we work hard to make it a success. We bring in Namibian beef, and fish – frozen kabeljou (cod) and rock lobster – that has to be brought in ice from Frankfurt by special courier so it does not spoil. We find boerewors made locally not far from Berlin and Namibia Breweries supplies us with a few crates of Windhoek Lager.

I phone the wives of some of the embassy officials, and the Namibian women diplomats at the embassy and ask for their help.

'I thought we could all work together at the residence to prepare the food,' I say, 'the cooking will mostly be done at the restaurant.'

The women come the day before the brunch and we crowd into the kitchen, peel beans, strip mealies of their leaves, chop spinach, cut the boerewors into portions and prepare tomato and onion sauce for the meat. I go into the sitting room to talk to Peter about the drinks and overhear the conversations going on in the kitchen, in English, Oshiwambo, OtjiHerero, Khoe-Khoe-Gowab and Afrikaans.

'Listen,' I say to him. 'It's just like being back in Namibia.'

Lambert's own personal contribution is fried plantain, a dish common in Central and West Africa (he comes from Benin). It's not a Namibian dish, but Peter and I love it, so we agree to include it.

Over 400 people come to the brunch. Peter and I are slightly late. The information sent out says that it will start at 11.30 but we can't believe that people will be there on the dot. When we arrive at 11.40 there's already a queue to get in, and more people quickly come and fill up the restaurant.

We invite a Namibian musician, Willie, to come over for the event from Sweden where he's is currently based. He's joined by Patricia, a Namibian woman singer who's spending six months at a music college in the south of Germany, and Ees, who was at school with Perivi. Although he's a white, German-speaking Namibian, his chosen style is Namibian township kwaito music.

We also host a Namibia Day reception in the Rotes Rathaus, the red town hall in Berlin, where 700 people come – businessmen and women, diplomats, politicians, and Namibians. The Minister for Economic Cooperation and Development, Heidemarie Wieczorek-Zeul, is also there and we feel honoured to have her at the event. Lambert again organises the preparation and cooking of Namibian food, although this time it's mostly small beef kebabs and other finger food.

The presence of the Minister at our Namibia Day reception highlights the special relationship felt between Namibia and Germany. It also reflects the ongoing issue that we cannot escape: that of the atrocities committed by German troops in Namibia in 1904-08. It was Minister Wieczorek-Zeul who apologised on behalf of the German Government for these atrocities, at the Ohamakari commemoration in 2004.

Peter carries the history of those days with him personally. His Aunt Maria, who raised him, was a survivor. Her older sister was held in one of the concentration camps in Windhoek, and then taken to work on one of the German farms. Peter himself grew up in Okandjira, the site of one of the main battles with the Germans. There are graves of German soldiers at the base of one of the nearby hills.

Many children were born of Herero mothers and German fathers during the German colonial period, most of them the outcome of forced, not consensual relations. There are light-skinned Hereros and members of other African communities in central and southern Namibia, who show that ancestry. Luther's mother's father was German. His mother's skin was pale except for her face and hands that were exposed to the sun; her hair was long and straight, and Luther talks of how he and his siblings loved to touch it. Peter's maternal great-grandfather was also German.

At the time of Namibia's Independence, the Herero Chief Kuaima Riruako launched a legal challenge to the German state and to German companies that had operated in Namibia at the turn of the twentieth century, in the early years of German rule. He filed a case in the US federal court seeking reparations from them for what he termed the genocide of thousands of Herero who were killed and enslaved during their uprising against German rule. Preliminary hearings established that it was possible to make such a claim for reparations for war crimes committed overseas, under an old Act from the late eighteenth century.

Not surprisingly, the terms 'genocide' and 'reparations' are not liked in Germany, because they have such legal significance and raise questions about who would be eligible for reparations, how to identify them, and how to quantify their suffering. However, following the apology, the German Government has offered €20 million to Namibia in a 'Special Initiative' aimed at helping present-day members of all communities of central and southern Namibia who suffered under German rule. This is in addition to development aid that is already given to Namibia by Germany.

Consultations between the Namibian and German Governments, and with the affected communities, are underway to identify socio-economic projects that will benefit those communities: water provision, gardening and small-scale agricultural projects will be the first to be implemented.

'What do you think about the Special Initiative?' I ask Peter when he brings me up to date about it.

'It's a gesture of goodwill,' he tells me, 'and welcome development assistance.' He pauses. 'But it's a German initiative. It's not based on a proper needs assessment and I don't know if it will really address the concerns of our communities for recognition of what they suffered, and some sort of compensation linked to that.'

'It sounds like a lot of money,' I say. 'But the Memorial to the Murdered Jews of Europe is supposed to have cost about €25 million, and that's nothing to do with actual reparations. And I read the other day about the amounts of money being spent renovating old buildings in Berlin. They're ten times that sum, or more.'

'Really?' he asks. 'If that's the cost of renovation, what is the price of reconciliation?'

The US court case is waiting for further action on the Namibian side, but Chief Riruako also tabled a motion in the Namibian National Assembly declaring Germany's atrocities 'genocide', and calling for reparations for the affected communities. It won unanimous support and was passed in late 2006.

Now, in June 2007, a similar motion is introduced in the German Parliament by the Left Party – the coalition between the left wing of the Social Democratic Party (SDP) and the remnants of the Socialist People's Party of the GDR. The remaining SDP is angry with its left-wing members who broke away to join the Left Party, and want nothing to do with them or their motion on Namibia. Peter is advised by some German friends not to get involved. Yet Chief Riruako is invited by the Left Party to be present at the time the motion is debated and he comes to Berlin with a delegation from the Herero Committee on Reparations.

The Chief, his wife, who wears traditional Herero dress and *otjikaeva* headdress, the head of the Herero Committee on Reparations – a woman who also wears Herero dress and *otjikaeva* – and other members of the delegation, plus staff from the embassy, Peter and I, go to the VIP visitors' balcony inside the German Parliament Chamber for the debate. We create quite a stir as we walk up the stairs of the Reichstag and through its corridors, with tourists, parliamentary staff and MPs stopping to look at us.

The Reichstag has been renovated using modern styles and materials in addition to the old. Inside are elements retained from all four powers that were in charge of Berlin after the War: the Soviet Union, Britain, France and the USA. Soviet graffiti dated May 1945, scratched on the inside walls, reflect the moment Berlin fell to the Allies; they have not been scrubbed away.

A new glass dome, designed by British architect Norman Foster, crowns the building. In its centre is a mirrored glass cone reflecting light down into the Chamber of the Parliament. It's open at the top, creating an outlet for hot air and an inlet of fresh air, beautiful and symbolic at the same time.

The VIP balcony seems to float in the air, suspended under the glass dome, facing the chair of the Speaker of the Parliament and the German eagle behind. We take our seats and look down on the MPs below. The presiding officer opens the proceedings and acknowledges our presence; the parliamentarians clap in greeting.

'Just being here feels like a small victory,' I whisper to Peter from my seat in the row behind him. He is in the front row with the Chief.

The motion is tabled by an MP of Turkish descent, Hueseyin Aydin. It asks the German government to accept its 'historical responsibility' and to acknowledge the right of the Hereros and Namas to reparations due to the genocide committed by the German troops. The debate is short. There is a consensus that terrible things took place and reminders of the Special Initiative. The motion is then referred to the Foreign Affairs Committee of the German Parliament for further discussions.

Two days later, the Chief and his delegation go home and report to President Pohamba, the Ministry of Foreign Affairs and other leaders of the affected communities. Peter proposes to take the matter up with the new Speaker of the Namibian Parliament, Dr Theo-Ben Gurirab, who is due to come to Berlin soon on an official visit to his counterpart, the President of the German Bundestag, Dr Norbert Lammert.

The new Speaker is another old friend of ours and an old colleague of Peter's. When Peter was Representative in London, he was SWAPO Representative at the UN in New York. When he and his African American wife, Joan, come to Berlin, it is with a multi-party delegation of five Namibian MPs, two parliamentary assistants and their translator. Peter goes to Frankfurt to meet the delegation at the airport, and accompanies them to Dresden. There they meet the President of the State Parliament, tour the city and visit the Opera. The following day, they proceed to Meissen and tour the cathedral and the porcelain factory there, and then come on to Berlin. I go to the hotel in central Berlin where they will be staying, to be part of the reception party for them. I introduce myself to the hotel manager who is waiting for them, and we stand at the end of the red carpet laid out for them, as they arrive in their official convoy, with police motorbike outriders.

The Speaker and MPs have meetings with the President of the Bundestag, political parties and non-governmental organisations. The outcome of the Left Party's motion on Namibia is discussed, and they agree that the two parliaments should find a way to discuss the matter between them and engage in further dialogue on the matter.

Joan has a separate programme, which I have been involved in planning, and on which I accompany her. We attend a rehearsal at one of the Berlin Opera houses of a performance of 'Die Fledermaus' and are amused at the translator's rendition of it into English as 'Batman'. We go to the Altes Museum to see the Egyptian collection, including an exhibition of ancient jewellery and the famous bust of Nefertiti.

'I wanted you to see this,' I tell Joan when we get to the bust. 'I've been here already and I love it.'

'I've seen ones like this in Cairo as well,' Joan tells me.

'Standing there beside Nefertiti, you look very like her,' I say. Joan has short hair wrapped in an African cloth, a long graceful neck, similar colouring and an elegance and style that match what we can see of Nefertiti from the bust.

I also arrange for us to visit the Ethnology Museum near us in Dahlem where there's a wonderful exhibition of African Art that looks at different themes across African cultures, countries and historical periods. It shows how styles have differed in many ways, exploding some of the myths about static African art, and showing how twentieth-century modern artists like Picasso drew on African art.

After Joan, Theo-Ben and the delegation have returned to Namibia, we discover that there are skulls in the basement of the Ethnology Museum. They include skulls of Hereros and Namas killed during the 1904-08 resistance to German rule, and taken to Germany for so-called scientific research.

'It makes me feel quite sick,' I tell Peter when I hear about it.

'I'm familiar with that feeling,' he replies.

Late in June, I'm taken ill one night. I go to bed feeling deeply tired but assuming that a good night's sleep is all I need. Then I wake at midnight to the phone ringing. I reach out to pick up the receiver on the phone by the bed, and answer sleepily. It's Perivi.

'Hello my dear,' I say. 'Everything alright?' It's unusual to get a call from Perivi since we usually phone him.

'Everything's fine,' he says. 'I was just thinking of you and wanted to talk to you.'

I switch on the bedside lamp and sit up. Peter is not with me; he left for Frankfurt earlier that day for a meeting between the European Union and the African, Caribbean and Pacific countries. I reach for the pillows from Peter's side of the bed to add to my own, and plump them up behind me. Perivi and I chat for a while but as we do so I start to feel dizzy, and I rest my head back on the pillows.

Perivi asks me for the address of someone in the family and I get up to find my address book. I walk into the family room but the dizziness gets worse, I feel disorientated and my breathing is very shallow.

'I'll have to call you back tomorrow, Perivi,' I say. 'I'm just too tired now.' I end the call and go back and sit on the side of the bed. Dull pains start across my chest and do not stop, and I realise that I need medical assistance.

I put on one of my African dresses over my nightie, pick up my ID and medical aid card and the small bag of medication that I keep in the bedside drawer, and go downstairs to find the emergency number. I phone for an ambulance. The pain is tight across my chest but I feel calm because I know help will come. I go down to the basement and knock on the door to wake Lambert.

'I'm not feeling well,' I tell him.

'Shall I call an ambulance?' he asks.

'I've already done that,' I reply.

Lambert puts on a gown and comes upstairs. He sits me down on one of the sofas and goes to get me a glass of water. When he brings it back, I don't want to drink it. The pain has intensified and I find it difficult to breathe.

In a strange detached state, I wonder why dying has to be so painful. Then two paramedics arrive. Lambert lets them in and they come over to me. They test my blood pressure, listen to my heart, and ask me questions. I try to explain my medical history briefly, although I don't feel like speaking at all.

'We think you might be having a heart attack,' they tell me and they prepare a syringe.

'What's in that?' I ask.

'Morphine.'

'I can't take any opiates,' I tell them in a daze. 'I've had morphine before and it crashes my blood pressure. I don't want it, please.'

They put the syringe away, stand either side of me, lift me up from the chair and walk with me to the front door and down the few steps. They put me into a wheelchair and into the ambulance, and rush me to a nearby hospital. I'm wheeled into an emergency room and plugged onto monitors to see what my heart is doing. I will be safe in their care, I think, and I start to let go.

A little later, I open my eyes to see Lambert and Edward standing beside me, looking worried.

'We phoned Ambassador to tell him you're in hospital, Madame,' says Edward.

'Thank you.'

'How are you feeling?' he asks me.

By now, my symptoms have eased and the pains across my chest have subsided.

'A little better,' I say. They stay with me for ten minutes and then leave.

The doctor on duty comes in.

'We've looked at the record of your heartbeat and we don't think it was a heart attack after all,' he tells me. 'But we want to keep you in hospital overnight.'

I'm taken to a small, two-bed room; the other bed is occupied but the patient is asleep.

In the morning, the cardiology team come to talk to me and take my medical history. I go right back to 2003 and the time my pacemaker was put in. I tell them about the episodes of tachycardia in Brussels, the pains across my chest after coming to Berlin and how I felt the night before.

'What medication are you taking?' they ask. I show them my bag of medicine and they note it down.

'This is a high dose of beta-blocker,' one of them says. 'If I took that much it would knock me out.' He's a lot taller than I am, and thicker set.

He leaves the room and comes back again half an hour later.

'We've discussed your condition and we think the attack was probably caused by dangerously low blood pressure,' he says, 'perhaps connected to your medication. We'd like to keep you in for a few days to do some tests.'

They wheel me down the corridor for a chest X-ray and heart sonar and back to my room. The other occupant is a middle-aged woman and we introduce ourselves to each other in a mixture of German and English. The door opens and Peter walks in. He comes to my bedside and takes my hand.

'Sweetheart, I'm sorry I wasn't here,' he says. 'How are you doing now?'

I hold onto his hand and tears come into my eyes.

'They're looking after me really well,' I tell him. 'The hospital is one of the top heart clinics in the world, or so I'm told by the doctors. I'm hopeful they may find out more about what's going on with my heart.'

'Perivi and Isabel send their love,' Peter tells me, 'and Uanaingi. I spoke to them all.'

'How are they?' I ask.

'They're fine. Naturally, they're worried about you.'

There follows the most thorough series of investigations I've ever had. Not content with the past diagnosis that I had a virus in my heart, the cardiologists do a range of tests to see what the condition of my heart is. There are blood tests, ECGs at rest and while exercising (on a stationary bicycle). Three different catheters (on three separate occasions) are inserted to check my arteries, the pressure in my heart at rest and while exercising, and to do a biopsy, in which they take a microscopic sample of my heart tissue to examine it.

Some of the results come while I'm still in hospital.

'The pressure in your heart is too high,' the doctors tell me one day on their early morning rounds.

'That describes what I've felt doing exercise,' I tell them. 'Thank you. Now I know I wasn't imagining the difficulty.'

I have to wait longer for the result of the biopsy and, after four days, I leave the hospital and go home.

When the results come through, Peter and I go to see the chief cardiologist in his consulting room.

'The biopsy confirms that there's a virus in your heart,' the cardiologist tells me. It's a common virus linked to colds and flu.

'What's the prognosis?' I ask him.

'An infection of the heart normally causes ongoing deterioration, either rapidly or slowly,' he says, looking me straight in the eye. This is what I had always feared.

'However, there's also some inflammation,' he says, 'and that shows that your heart is fighting the infection. I want to change and intensify your medication to help your heart fight the infection. Then we'll do further tests in a year's time to see what progress you've made and whether some other treatment needs to be considered.'

I start to feel better with the new medication but the strength of it overwhelms me at times. I lose my balance and fall heavily as I come out of a restaurant with Peter and Uazuvara, when he's on one of his visits to Berlin. I turn to talk to them as we go down a few steps to the pavement, and I lose my balance and tip over backwards. I feel myself falling away from them and know that I won't be able to turn round in time to put my hands out to break the fall. I hit the ground on the left side of my chest and lie there, winded, while Peter and Uazuvara jump down to pick me up.

'No, please, wait...' I say. It really hurts where I've fallen and I go to the hospital the next morning to get an X-ray and to ask them to check my spleen. Fortunately everything is clear and I recover over the next two weeks.

A month later, I fall up the steps at a reception given by the British Ambassador. This time, the fall is not as hard. I pick myself up, stand by the wall at the side for a while to gather myself, and then continue up the steps to join the reception. Peter holds my arm anxiously and everyone around is very solicitous. I just feel very foolish. After this, Peter starts to hold my arm whenever we are facing steps; that, I don't mind.

Earlier in the year, before I went into hospital, I travelled with Aicha to Norway, for the confirmation of Uazuvara and Bente's younger daughter, Nora. Almost all children get confirmed in Norway; it's both a religious and a social celebration, a transition to maturity. Nora's confirmation was held on her 15th birthday, in May. It was also the anniversary of Mosé's funeral. He was one of her godfathers and his death blighted her birthday last year.

Nora's other Namibian godparents came and her godmother, Karee, wore a golden, tawny brown traditional Herero dress and *otjikaeva*, which fitted in well with the traditional Norwegian dresses worn by Bente and some of the other women. Nora was also dressed in traditional Norwegian costume – her first – made by Bente in between all her work commitments. It had a long, full black skirt, a white blouse with full sleeves and small collar, pinned at the throat, a little red waistcoat and long white embroidered apron. Bente wore the same costume, with a thin red band round her short hair. Uazuvara wore a dark suit with white shirt and silver tie, in contrast to the casual shirts he usually wears.

A whole group of teenage girls was being confirmed at the same time and Nora's girlfriends were also in traditional costumes, differing slightly from each other, depending on the area of Norway their families came from.

After the service in a large, cold Lutheran church, family and friends walked through an icy wind to the new International School Bente helped to establish and where she is the principal. We sat down for a meal at a U-shaped arrangement of tables in the school hall. Bente's parents were there, her brothers and their wives or partners, children of varying ages, aunts and uncles and close friends. The Namibian and Norwegian flags hung on the wall behind the head table.

There were gifts and speeches honouring Nora. Karee gave her traditional Namibian gifts – a carved wooden cup and *onduzu*, a container made out of a tortoise shell, traditionally used for *otjizumba* powder (made from a sweet smelling tree and used by Herero women). Ida, in grey trousers, black and white top and black loose-knitted shawl, presented a slide show of photos of Nora, looking proudly at her little sister but managing to make some witty jokes about her as well.

'You should have seen the smile on Nora's face throughout it all,' I told Peter as I described the event to him back in Berlin. 'She was empowered by the love of family and friends, the attention they gave her, the things they said about her.'

Perivi was confirmed in Namibia, when he was 15, and we threw a party for him too. I made a photo album for him of his life and told him we would have to treat him more as an adult now that he was growing up. Isabel has not been confirmed. We didn't have a church in Brussels that we went to; nor do we yet in Berlin. Despite my religious searching and my quest for faith, I'm wary of organised religion, especially in the current international climate where men of war claim that God is on their side.

After Nora's confirmation party, however, I want to do something similar for Isabel. She left home before we expected her to, necessitated by our move to Berlin, and I've spent the past year thinking that I hadn't said enough, hadn't taught her to sew or to cook, hadn't guided her enough for her adult life. So we plan a party in Berlin for her. She was baptised in the United Church of Christ at Yale University in the USA when she was ten months' old. It's a self-proclaimed open and affirming church, and we call her party an Affirmation Party.

Shortly before the party takes place, Peter decides we need to add a traditional Herero element to it. He says that if Isabel were at home, she would be taken to the village by the women in the family and be given her first Herero dress and *otjikaeva*, so we order one to be made for her. Uanaingi takes on the task and she and I send each other cell phone messages about colours and sizes, measurements from shoulder to waist and waist to floor; I have to measure some of Isabel's clothes in her cupboard and estimate the right size. We tell Uanaingi to courier it to us to make sure it will be with us on the day but, better than that, the Namibian Foreign Minister flies through Frankfurt the week before the party and Peter has to meet him there. So the Foreign Minister ends up being the courier, and he brings Isabel's dress, three glorious lacy petticoats and the *otjikaeva*, tied and ready to put on.

We hold the party at the residence. The date has been chosen to fit in with Perivi's mid-term break and he flies over for a week to be with us. It's mid-September, the week before Isabel's 19th birthday, and we're lucky with the weather: it's still warm.

Isabel and five of her student friends drive over from Leiden. It's a six-hour journey and they leave after class on the Friday afternoon and arrive in the middle of the night. The following day, Isabel takes them round Berlin, and out with Aicha to a club on the Saturday night.

Some diplomatic friends we've grown close to come to the party on Sunday, as well as Laurie, head of the Cheetah Conservation Fund in Namibia, who is in Berlin at that time, but it's mostly family. Our Berlin family – embassy staff and their families, Aicha and her son Kara, Miriam and Matthias and their girls – and other Namibians living in Berlin, are there. My parents come to represent the UK family, and Isabel's favourite uncles Luther and Uazuvara are with us as well; her other favourite uncle was Mosé.

Isabel has pledged to continue the work of these her fathers – these men of the liberation struggle – and work to develop Namibia.

God is with us. Everyone gets here safely; the sun shines and we can sit inside or out. Miriam's girls run round the garden and play with Isabel and Perivi and Lambert's daughter Jesse. Lambert prepares a Namibian spread, chosen by Isabel, of Namibian beef brought over especially for the occasion, barbecued chicken pieces, boerewors, spinach sauce, potato salad and pap, and his speciality – fried plantain. We have Windhoek lager, French red wine, Italian and German white.

Before the party, I had written to friends and family around the world and asked them to send messages for Isabel, which I print and give her on the day.

Doris recalls Isabel climbing trees in her garden and always being full of happiness. Deedee affirms Isabel's active childhood and her gift for friendship. Mosé and Sandra's daughter Tjireya says how touched she is that Isabel feels inspired by Mosé: 'Though his sun has set, the radiance of his light is shining on through us,' she writes. My sister Helen recalls 'the joy of sharing you as my borrowed daughter from far off lands'. Helen's son Antonio congratulates Isabel on starting 'as the cute, funny cousin who's now turned into a beautiful, intelligent and savvy woman'. My brother John writes, 'Life is a precious gift from God' and quotes the Old Testament prophet Micah: '*Act justly and love mercy and walk humbly with your God*'. Her Namibian godparents Kapee and Tate Tommy give her a cow and calf (to be held on their farm in Namibia on her behalf).

Peter and I pay tribute to her, as does Uazuvara.

'Isabel, you know how proud we are of you, and how much we love you,' Peter tells her. 'We admire you for all that you've achieved.

You've embarked on your studies and your independent journey now, and we wish you well and want to remind you that you have our ongoing support.'

'For 17 years, Isabel said she would never leave home,' I tell the assembled guests. 'Then one day she was suddenly ready. She found the place she wanted to go to, and off she went, to study in Leiden. I sometimes say that this was a sudden departure and suggest that Isabel wasn't prepared for it. It's taken me this year, though, to realise that it was me who wasn't ready to let her go.'

I give Isabel a photo album I have made of her life so far.

'You are brave and determined, observant and thoughtful,' I tell her. 'You face challenges with courage. You see things clearly and you see things through. You are charming and beautiful, loving and funny. We celebrate you.'

Then I gather together the Namibian women and we go upstairs with Isabel to give her the dress. It's a complete surprise for her and she starts to weep, saying how it makes her feel fully accepted as part of the Herero community. The dress is pale green with a border pattern of stylised leaves and flowers in green, beige and pink at the bottom of the skirt, and a turquoise swirl. The colours suit her and the *otjikaeva* fits perfectly. We gather her loose curls backwards, put the *otjikaeva* on top of her head and pin it on with hairclips. We take her downstairs and one of the Namibian women ululates as we descend. Isabel glides into the room, smiling radiantly, and everyone grabs their cameras to take photos.

We send one of the photos of us all, with Isabel in her Herero dress, to the newspapers in Namibia and Sandy phones the next Sunday to say she's just seen it. She has been mourning her father, who died a month ago in his sleep, in Zimbabwe, and she tells us that seeing the photo is like a sudden unexpected visit from us, cheering her heart. Her father was given a Hindu cremation as was her mother, but there was no muslin available in which to wrap the body, because of all the shortages. So Sandy told her sister in the UK to bring over a Superman duvet, which she did, and their father was wrapped in that and cremated. His ashes were gathered and scattered in the same place that Sandy's mother's had been.

When we print the photos of Isabel's party, I look at the ones of her and Perivi playing with Miriam's children, and I see their warmth and care. I know they will be wonderful parents when their time comes. Who could ask for more than to see these two beautiful young people grow and share the love that we, and others, have given them? However, I know that if I am not physically here to see that, I will be in their arms as they embrace their children, in their voices as they sing to them or tell them stories, in their hearts as they feel for them.

The month after Isabel's party, I go to spend a weekend with Bente at her parent's cabin in the Norwegian mountains. I accepted her invitation with delight and some trepidation because Bente is so fit and active.

'I'm worried about climbing the hills,' I told her.

'Well, we'll take it gently,' she said.

I fly to Oslo and overnight with Patji and the family, then go on by bus the next day to meet up with Bente. It's October and in Berlin the weather is still mild and sunny; in Norway, it's much colder.

The wood cabin perches on the side of a hill, surrounded on two sides by fir trees, with an outside tap by a well for our water supply. Grass grows on the roof and provides extra insulation from the cold. There are two tiny bedrooms with bunk beds in, and an open kitchen, living and eating area. The cabin is cold from being empty for some time and we make up a wood fire and turn on the electric heaters full blast as well. During the night, the temperatures drop well below zero and we put on our clothes and huddle under all the blankets we can find.

The next day, the air is crisp but cold and the sun is out.

'Let's go for a short walk,' Bente says. I put on tights, two pairs of trousers, a thick sweater and a padded jacket to protect myself from the cold.

Bente leads me past the other cabins scattered about the hills. We go further than I expect, and higher too.

'See the ski runs that we use in winter,' Bente points out across the valley.

She turns to me: 'It's so nice to have you here, my dear. This is such an important place to me. I'm glad that you can see it.'

We walk on a little further, up a gentle rise. She looks up the hill.

'You can see a lake from the top,' she tells me.

'I don't know how far up I can go,' I say.

Bente leads me along paths that don't ascend too steeply and we keep stopping so that I can rest. Dry brownish heather and bracken cover the mountain, broken by patches of rock. Small, bare silver birch trees are silhouetted against the blue sky.

Bente walks on ahead of me while I stop to look at crystal ice formations in the undergrowth. I move on slowly to join her, looking at the path rather than the view. The land starts to level out. I bypass some rocks on a little path and suddenly, without my realising it, I come to the summit. The sight in front of us is stunning – a huge lake of the brightest blue and the snow-capped Hardangervidda mountains in the distance on the other side. I can't believe that I have made it to the top.

I return to Berlin encouraged by my achievement and decide to go ahead with a visit to Namibia I want to make. It's a year since I was there and I long to go again. I want to see friends and family and do some research for a novel I've been thinking about for years.

I decide to time a visit to coincide with Deedee's 50th birthday in February 2008, and I fly in a few days beforehand. I stay with Deedee for a few days, sleeping in her guest room at the bottom of her garden, completely quiet except for the sounds of the birds in the thorn trees. I have no responsibilities, and plenty of time to catch up with Deedee and think about my novel. Even the series of steps that lead up from the guest room to her main living area and balcony do not daunt me as much as they used to.

Deedee throws a birthday party at home with a Moroccan theme, including shishas on the balcony and a Moroccan meal. About 50 of us gather to celebrate and congratulate her. Tables and chairs are laid out in the downstairs room and Michael stands up to welcome us all. He makes a few jokes about Deedee, wishes her Happy Birthday, and others follow with their own contributions. I stand up.

'I'd like to say something about what Deedee means to me,' I say. 'She's a very positive person. She's full of encouragement. If you have a problem and ask for Deedee's advice, she'll ask you what you want to do. And whatever you decide, she will tell you that you've made the right decision.' I pause while people laugh. 'But Deedee is also very tenacious,' I say. 'She doesn't give up. She didn't give up on me five years ago when she could see that I needed medical help. She made sure that I got to the doctor.' I pause again to gather my composure. 'Thank you Deedee.'

We all toast her and then she responds. She looks at her women friends around her. 'I've been thinking about what someone said to me tonight about all these intelligent women in Windhoek,' she says. 'So I'd like to raise a toast: Here's to intelligent women and good-looking men!'

'Yay!' says Sandy. 'Excellent!' We raise our glasses.

After we've eaten, I join Jane and Helao on the terrace. The evening is cool and Jane has wrapped a thick shawl round her shoulders. She looks pale and drawn. She's just come back from her brother-in-law's funeral in the UK. He died suddenly, soon after they were all gathered together for her father's 100th birthday. She arrived back in Windhoek from the birthday celebration to be given the news, and had to turn around and go straight back to England for the funeral.

I move on from Deedee's to stay for a few days with Sandy, and Peter joins me there, coming home for meetings of his own. We haven't seen much of the Namibian family for a long time and it's good to spend time with Uanaingi, Diana, Utaa and Penaani. We visit other relatives as well, including Eva, one of Peter's sisters, who is very ill in hospital after an operation for breast cancer.

I invite Deedee and Michael, Hugo, Jane and Helao to join Sandy and Ted, Peter and me for a meal at Sandy's house. I organise delivery of salads and chicken dishes from our favourite delicatessen, and buy red and white wine and beer for the men. For Peter's and my benefit, Sandy shows the video of her recent production 'The Lion Roars', co-written by her and Jackson Kaujeua, who sang at my 50th birthday party, and whose life story and music the show depicts. We talk about getting the show to Berlin under the cultural exchange partnership programme.

But I have another, very specific, reason for bringing everyone together.

'Here's the thing,' I say when we've nearly finished the meal. 'I've been writing.' I pause. 'I've been writing about Namibia, and about all of you.' I laugh nervously. 'I did warn you,' I say to Sandy, Deedee and Jane, and take a drink from my glass of wine.

'I started to write this story in Brussels,' I continue. 'I felt uprooted from my Namibian home, and shaken by Isobel's death, my being ill, and Sandy being ill. I wanted to answer the question, "What happened to us all?"' I pause. 'But when I became engaged in the writing process I began to realise that this was also a story about my own journey.'

I stop, overcome by emotion. Peter puts his hand out and covers mine. I take a deep breath.

'I want to continue,' I say. 'But I need to know what you think about me writing about you. So I'd like to show you the draft and if you'd rather I didn't do this, I won't.'

I give them each a ring-bound typescript of what I've written so far, wrapped in a plastic bag; I don't want them to start looking at it now.

'Wow, Janie!' exclaims Jane.

I talk to each of them in turn over the next week as they look at what I've written.

'I'm honoured by what you write, Jane,' Deedee says, 'but it's rather strange, reading about yourself.'

'Is is truthful?' I ask her.

'Yes, I think so.'

'Is this really how people see me?' Jane asks, and then tells me that there are one or two factual details she'd like to discuss. I go to her house to talk to her and Helao about them.

I arrange to meet Sandy at the wine bar to find out what she thinks.

'You've described me as politically incorrect!' she announces as soon as she arrives.

'Would you rather I didn't?' I ask.

'Deedee says it's a compliment,' she tells me.

'Maybe it is,' I say, and take a drink of my wine.

'I tried to write it as a novel,' I explain, 'but the sequence of some of the events didn't seem believable. I tried to write it with pseudonyms to protect you all, but Namibia's such a small society that we all know each other and it didn't make sense to do so.'

We talk about it for a while but she has to leave for a rehearsal at her theatre. I leave the wine bar with her and we walk together to our cars, and give each other a kiss to say goodbye. Sandy jumps into her car and starts to drive off slowly. She winds down the window, waves her arm high out of it and shouts to the world:

'I'm politically incorrect!'

Hugo takes the copy of my transcript with him to the airport and reads much of it there because his flight is delayed for hours. I hear from him later in an email:

'Reading the parts about Isobel's death was emotional... I was quite overwhelmed by the fact that someone else cared enough to remember the small details,' he writes. 'I found myself recalling the smells and sounds and faces that were so familiar in the Brasilian at the time. At one point I realised that the assistant manager at the time had since become manager of the airport coffee shop. As I looked up and made brief eye contact, I suddenly wondered whether she was recalling similar memories.'

Hugo's reading was made more poignant by the fact that he was waiting to fly to the funeral of his younger brother's wife, who died of heart failure at the age of 49, leaving two sons (19 and 20) and a 13-year-old daughter.

The novel I want to write looks at a young Namibian woman who comes of age at the time of Independence, and the choices she faces about whether to commit herself to community work in Namibia or pursue academic work abroad. The central character grows up in Walvis Bay, and I start my research for the book with interviews with people in Windhoek who grew up in this interesting coastal town. Walvis Bay is quite unlike Swakopmund. It's an industrial town, a port, with a history of trade union activity, and a highly politicised workforce who helped to build SWAPO. It's a town where Namibians from different communities have lived and worked together, despite the enforced separations under South African rule.

Peter and I travel to Walvis Bay for a long weekend, for me to do more interviews there. We drive across the desert to the coast and then south from Swakopmund along the stunning ocean road, with the grey-blue sea on one side and almost orange sand dune desert on the other. We go to Kuisebmund, the former township of Walvis Bay, with its strong history of resistance to South African rule and I interview a family there – two generations of women – who recall the 1970s and 1980s. I take photographs to remind myself of the geography and the look of the place, so that I can continue to work on the book when I'm back in Berlin.

'It's good to be doing something in Namibia again, not just visiting,' I tell Peter as we drive back to Windhoek. 'I want to come back again later in the year, maybe in six months' time, to continue with my research.'

'Really?'

'Yes. In fact, I feel ready to return to my Namibian home now.'

He looks at me. 'But we've got another two years in Berlin.'

Soon after we get back to Berlin, Peter receives a phone call to tell him that his sister Eva has died in hospital in Windhoek.

'I'm glad we went to see her,' he says. She had thought she was dying but the doctors did not tell us what her prospects were.

Peter travels home for the funeral and comes back to Berlin again a few days later. The afternoon of the day he gets back, there's a phone call from State House, saying that the President wants to meet him – they thought he was still in Namibia. So Peter arranges to go back to Namibia again, for a meeting with the President.

Because of the nature of the call, the fact that no subject was given for the meeting, and that a Cabinet Minister had recently died in a car accident and not been replaced, we wonder whether some sort of offer to Peter might be forthcoming. We're lucky to have a few days before the meeting to talk about the implications.

'I'm still in the middle of things here,' Peter says. 'I don't feel I've finished.'

'But it would be lovely for you,' I respond. 'It would be the perfect step in terms of your career, your life's work for Namibia.'

'Well, we don't know yet if that's what the call is about,' Peter cautions.

After he leaves for Windhoek, I try not to think about it in case it doesn't come about.

While Peter is back in Windhoek and I'm waiting to hear from him, I get a call from Perivi.

'I want to go home,' he says. 'It's time. I want to go home now and make films.'

'What do you mean?' I ask.

'Someone asked me the other day who I want to make films for,' he tells me, 'and I realised that I've only ever wanted to make films for Namibia, for Namibians.'

'Well, yes, but you can do that in good time,' I say. 'What about your course?'

'I've learnt what I need to,' he says. 'It's time for me to go home. Can you get me a ticket? I don't want to be in Los Angeles any longer.' There's an unexpected urgency to his voice that stops me from arguing against his request.

'I don't know,' I tell Perivi. 'Honestly, I don't know. Let me talk to Daddy and I'll call you tomorrow.' I don't want to tell him that Peter is in Namibia as we speak, but if Peter is going to be reassigned, everything will change.

The next day, Peter phones to give me his news. I pick up the call in the kitchen. When I hear his voice, I sit down at the small kitchen table and look out at the street through the window. Luckily, Lambert is not around.

'Sweetheart,' he says. 'Are you there?'

'Yes,' I reply. 'What happened? Have you had your meeting yet?' My heart is beating fast.

'Yes,' he pauses. 'I've just come from State House. I've been offered the post of Director General of the National Planning Commission. It's a full Cabinet position.'

'Wow!' I say. 'It's really happening.'

'Yes.' He pauses. 'I've already been sworn in.'

'Wow!' I say again. 'It's so fast.'

'It's part of a wider Cabinet reshuffle,' Peter explains. 'They were just waiting for me before making it public.'

'Congratulations,' I say. My mind is buzzing.

'Thank you. I can't talk much now. I've got to go into various meetings to do with my new position and I'll be back in Berlin at the end of the week.'

'When are you supposed to start?' I ask.

'Well, I've already started. But I'll have to come and hand over in Berlin.'

When Perivi phones again that evening, I ask him how he's feeling.

'The same,' he says. 'I don't want to be here anymore. I need to go home.'

'Well, it seems as if we're all being pulled back home,' I say, and I tell him about Peter's appointment.

'I'll come via Berlin and help you pack,' Perivi says.

In one month, Peter winds up his work in Berlin, says his farewells, and returns to Namibia. Perivi arrives from the USA and accompanies him home. Lambert, Janet, and I do the packing in a great rush. Miriam comes to help.

Isabel cancels her intended summer school courses to be part of the family's return, and joins in the packing.

'I need to be back in Southern Africa again after being in Europe for four years,' she tells me.

Before we go, I return to see the cardiologist to tell them that I'm leaving and ask what I should tell the doctors at home. They do more tests that show that my heart function has improved. Then they do a second biopsy. A week later, I go to get the results.

'The virus has gone,' the cardiologist tells me, with some surprise. My heart is finally free of infection.

Isabel and I leave two weeks after Peter and Perivi. We are seen off at Berlin's Tegel airport by diplomats from our embassy and from other SADC embassies. We travel business class, looked after as important dignitaries by the protocol people of the German Foreign Affairs Ministry. One of the embassy drivers has already driven to Frankfurt with our luggage – a large collection of suitcases – but we fly there. We're escorted through passport and other controls, and installed in our own VIP lounge in Frankfurt while in transit – the wife and daughter of an outgoing ambassador, now Cabinet Minister. We transfer to Air Namibia for the flight home and are greeted by the crew and given glasses of champagne. I'm astonished that we got everything done and have made it this far. I feel very tired but excited too. Isabel is humming.

The protocol relaxes after we leave Germany and arrive back in Namibia. We're met by Peter and two drivers, who load all our suitcases and boxes into two cars and take us to a small government guest house where we'll stay for two months until the tenants move out of our house.

The grand days of Berlin, the residence with its mirrored rooms and silk wall coverings, are past. The support staff, who bought new light bulbs and changed them, called the plumber, cooked the food, washed and ironed the clothes, are left behind.

We are back 'at home' but not yet at home, readjusting, reconnecting, going round to find phone and internet connections, and a second-hand car for me. We need to buy blankets to add to the duvets provided in the guest house as it's low-lying and extremely cold. We need towels, pillows, buckets, cleaning materials and a vacuum cleaner. There are no more smart lunches for me, no leisurely receptions. I live in old trousers and T-shirts, cleaning the temporary house to make it liveable in. Once the tenants have moved out of our own house, I turn my attention to that, guiding the decorators, choosing paint colours, getting quotes on curtains and garden restoration.

For previous moves in Namibia, whether from one house to another or one office to another or one shop to a new one, I had the practical support of Luther or Uazuvara, who were somehow always around at the right time. Now I rely on Isabel and our niece Eerike, to unpack the boxes of our books and other belongings that were packed in 2003 and left in storage.

Peter is immediately busy with his work at the National Planning Commission and out of the country often. His duties include coordinating donor aid to Namibia and this takes him to meetings around the world. It's a demanding post but he draws on his experience over the years. His earlier diplomatic work lobbying for SWAPO; his good contacts with people involved in development work; his management experience from the university; and his recent diplomatic work in Brussels and Berlin; all come together to prepare him for his new job.

Perivi jumps straight into writing scripts and planning films. He finds a short film competition with the theme of '18 years of Independence' – part of the cultural exchange programme between Berlin and Windhoek – and he works on a script to submit. He develops a concept of a three-scene film looking at relations between black and white within the setting of a small shop, and is one of three people whose films are selected for funding.

He picks up on a story from Peter's childhood of an occasion when Peter and his Aunt Maria went into a shop and were addressed very rudely by a young Afrikaans-speaking assistant. Peter's Aunt replied in German and when Peter asked her why she had done so, she told him that it was her way of showing the shop assistant, who could not understand German, that she didn't know everything.

This story inspires the first scene in Perivi's script, but he sets it in 1990, the year of Independence. The second scene is also based on a real experience shared with Perivi by someone he knows. He places it in the same shop, with the same shop assistant, about ten years' after Independence, when a black teenage customer reacts aggressively to the shop assistant's continued indifference. The third and final scene, set in the current day, shows an articulate, well-educated young black man who engages the shop assistant while questioning the rising prices of food.

'They're not my prices,' says the shop assistant. 'What do you expect me to do about it?'

'We could work together,' says the young man, and the script ends on that note.

Isabel catches up with old friends and drags me to the art shop to buy acrylic paint, brushes and canvasses. She spreads newspapers across the sitting room floor of the flat and paints a series of brightly coloured abstracts. She places a square brown wooden frame in the centre of one canvas, paints the background with a royal blue wash, and inside the square a deep orangey red. She drops small splashes of blue across the frame and the red paint within it, and red splashes across the blue. It's striking and the colours pulsate. I put it up in the entrance of our house when we move in and ask her if it has a title.

'Crossing Borders,' she says. 'It reflects my life.'

I walk down the Post Street Mall where my bookshop used to be. A new shopping centre has been built on one side, bustling with people buying clothes and household goods. I wonder if things would have worked out better for my bookshop if I had held on longer, and I jealously regard the window of the business that's based there now – selling printer ink and making a go of it.

In the time I've been away, the trees have grown larger and greener and their shade shelters shoppers and the sellers of art and crafts. One of the artists recognises me and greets me, asking where I've been all this time. It's a long story.

The arcade of cafés still buzzes with people but the Brasilian has changed hands and become a sports café. The new Brasilian, where I was drinking coffee with Sandy and Deedee when I heard from Peter that he had been appointed ambassador to Brussels, has been bought by the manager and renamed 'Café Brazza'. It's situated in a suburban shopping mall away from the heart of the city and the buzz that used to be my working environment.

It's at Café Brazza that Sandy, Deedee, and Jane meet now for Friday breakfasts. A new friend, Auriol, has joined them. A development consultant, originally from Britain, Auriol is married to a German-speaking Namibian and has lived in Namibia for 18 years. She's had significant input in the HIV/AIDS strategic plans and Deedee has worked with her a lot. Tall and very thin, with dark brown permed hair, she has a scientific background and is passionate about environmental issues.

On Friday mornings at 7.30, I take my place with them in this weekly ritual of friendship and support. Sandy and Deedee are still drinking skinny cappuccinos; Jane orders Earl Grey tea; Auriol has plain coffee. We order light cooked breakfasts.

'I want my egg hard, please, really hard,' says Deedee.

'Listen to her!' says Sandy. 'I won't have anything to eat, thanks. I've had porridge at home.'

'No onions for me, please,' I say.

'Who'll share a health breakfast with me?' Auriol asks.

'I will,' says Jane, 'as long as there aren't too many apples'. The waitress brings two small bowls of fruit and muesli with no apples in at all.

The conversation is dominated by the projects they're all busy with. I listen to them talking, deep in the details of their lives and work, and I wonder what I will become involved in now. For the first time in years, I can plan my future.

On the Sunday morning before Isabel is due to go back to The Netherlands for her next semester, I take her and Peter to St George's, the Anglican cathedral where Deedee's husband Michael is now Dean. It's the church where people prayed for me in 2003 when I was so ill. I've asked Michael if I can stand up and say something because I want to give thanks.

It's August and the light is hazy. The morning is still cool and I wear trousers and a jacket. The church is full and Deedee and Sandy are there. We sit in a pew in the middle of the church and I grow more nervous as the service progresses: I don't know if I will have the courage to say what I want to.

After the readings and the hymn for the collection, the new Associate Dean reads the notices. He calls for anyone who wants a special blessing for their birthday or anniversary, or for any special prayers, to come up to the altar rail. He signals me to come up.

'Come with me. I need your support,' I say to Peter and Isabel. I clutch the piece of paper on which I've written what I want to say, and we go up the aisle, climb the three steps towards the choir stalls, and turn to face the congregation. I take a deep breath.

'I've asked to say something today because I want to give thanks,' I say. 'I want to thank God for our safe return to Namibia and ask God's blessing on our work here and on Isabel as she returns to Europe to continue her studies.'

'I also want to give thanks to you, the congregation of St George's. When I was seriously ill with heart failure, you included me in your prayers for healing. I know that these prayers continued after we had gone to Brussels, and I thank you for them.'

I pause and take a deep breath to give myself the courage to continue.

'When we went to Brussels, I didn't think I would live very long,' I say. Peter reaches out and strokes my shoulder. Isabel starts to weep and I put my arm round her and hold her tightly.

I tell the congregation about the ups and downs with my health. I talk about reading the psalms in hospital in Brussels and getting such

299

comfort from them, and about my renewed faith. I tell them about the tests in Berlin and the recent biopsy that showed that the virus had gone from my heart. There's an audible gasp in response.

I give thanks for my healing – thanks to God, to the medical practitioners in four different countries who have helped me, and to the friends and family who have held me up with their love.

'Now I give thanks for this wonderful opportunity of a new start.' I say.

I conclude by reading the words of Psalm 103:

Bless the Lord, my soul;
My innermost heart, bless his holy name.
Bless the Lord, my soul,
And forget none of his benefits.
He pardons all my guilt
And heals all my suffering.
He rescues me from the pit of death
And surrounds me with constant love,
With tender affection.
He contents me with all good in the prime of life,
So that my youth is renewed like the eagle's.

Postcript

I read the proofs for *Undisciplined Heart* over the weekend of 21 March 2010, the twentieth anniversary of Namibian Independence. Celebrations were held across the country and thousands gathered at the Independence Stadium in Windhoek to see the swearing in of President Hifikepunye Pohamba for his second and final term. Heads of state and government, and former presidents from SADC countries, foreign ministers and representatives from Europe, Cuba, Russia and elsewhere, came to join our celebrations. Honours were given to the late ANC President O.R. Tambo, the late Angolan President Agostinho Neto, the late Tanzanian President Julius Nyerere, the President of the Congo Sassou Nguesso, former Foreign Minister of Angola Paulo Jorge, and the Belgian solidarity activist Paulette Pierson-Mathy, for their contributions to Namibia's struggle for independence.

In the appointment of a new administration, President Pohamba has moved Peter once again, to the National Assembly, where he has been sworn in as an MP, and has been nominated SWAPO Chief Whip, to coordinate government business in parliament along with the Speaker and the Prime Minister.

Perivi was busy preparing a film script for a sponsorship application. Three months previously, his second short film, 'Love is...' premiered at the cinema in Windhoek – the first Namibian film to do so. It portrays a young couple dealing with their relationship and finding space for their love even when their paths take them in different directions. The film was developed against the backdrop of widespread gender-based violence and shows a peaceful rather than violent resolution to conflict.

Isabel was in London, continuing with her degree in International Relations after a year doing Art at the University of Namibia, which had culminated in her first exhibition, 'Head to Toe', an exploration of colour and form – abstract paintings of the female form in acrylic on canvas.

As part of the independence celebrations, Sandy directed a powerful performance of dance and song at the National Theatre that captured and commemorated Namibia's history. It opened with the sound of South African helicopters bombing the Namibian settlement at Kassinga, in 1978, and took the audience through different periods of our history and the struggle for Independence. Jane and Helao's daughter Tuli, who had just completed a BA degree in African dance, danced in the show and assisted Sandy in the production.

Sandy's daughter, Brigit, had just completed a BA degree in Psychology (Hons), and joined Auriol as a research assistant for one of her consultancies. Sandy's son Ross has just got his BComm degree. Deedee's son Timmy was finishing his sports coaching diploma and working at the secondary school all our children went to in Windhoek. Jane's son had just finished there and was travelling round Australia during his gap year.

Helao went to the independence celebrations in his colonel's uniform and sat with other veterans. He was weak after suffering a slight stroke the month before, and almost two years fighting lymphoma, but his strength and determination are pulling him through.

Acknowledgements

Thanks are due to Modjaji, the rain queen, for showering me with her blessings. To Colleen Higgs, Modjaji's mother, for believing in this book while it was still being written. To the editor, Nella Freund, whose gentle but critical questioning, prodding and suggestions helped me to write better, opened up the story and doubled its length! And to my beloved husband Peter and children Isabel and Perivi, for their love and encouragement in all things.

The quotation from Birago Diop on page 256 is taken from Daniel and Olivier Föllmi (eds) *Origines: 365 Pensées de Sages Africains*, Editions de la Martinière, Paris, 2005, the entry for 11 January. The translation from the French is my own.

Other Modjaji Titles

Whiplash
by Tracey Farren

Invisible Earthquake
A Women's Journal Through Stillbirth
by Malika Ndlovu

Hester se Brood
Hester van der Walt

This Place I Call Home
by Meg Vandermerwe

The Thin Line
by Arja Salafranca

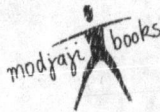

modjaji books

http://modjaji.book.co.za

www.ingramcontent.com/pod-product-compliance
Lightning Source LLC
Chambersburg PA
CBHW011828020426
42334CB00025B/2971